The Healthy Gut Handbook

Lose weight and boost your health with this simple 28-day plan

Justine Pattison

With a foreword by Professor Tim Spector, director of the British Gut Project

First published in Great Britain in 2017 by Seven Dials
This edition published in 2022 by Seven Dials
an imprint of The Orion Publishing Group Ltd
Carmelite House, 50 Victoria Embankment
London EC4Y 0DZ

An Hachette UK Company

3 5 7 9 10 8 6 4

A CIP catalogue record for this book is
available from the British Library.

ISBN (Mass Market Paperback) 978 1 4091 6692 4
ISBN (eBook) 978 1 4091 6693 1

Designed by Matt Inwood
Photographs by Cristian Barnett

Printed and bound by Clays Ltd, Elcograf S.p.A.

Every effort has been made to ensure that the information in this book is
accurate. The information will be relevant to the majority of people but
may not be applicable in each individual case, so it is advised that
professional medical advice is obtained for specific health matters.
Neither the publisher nor author accept any legal responsibility for any
personal injury or other damage or loss arising from the use or misuse of
the information in this book. Anyone making a change to their diet
should consult their GP, especially if pregnant, infirm, elderly or under 16.

www.orionbooks.co.uk

For my late father, John Pattison,
a man ahead of his time

Contents

PART THREE

The recipes 125

Foreword

by Professor Tim Spector

While on holiday a few years ago, I was struck down with a rare illness that suddenly left me with double vision, dizziness and high blood pressure. The symptoms resolved over the following months, but I was left needing a daily dosage of tablets and, crucially, was forced to re-evaluate my diet. As a practising doctor for over thirty years and the author of hundreds of research papers, many on obesity and weight, I considered myself well versed on nutrition and dieting. However, once I began to pick apart my seemingly healthy diet I realised that it was high in sugar, low in fat and – most startlingly – lacking in diversity. And I began a journey to discover the health repercussions that this lack of diversity can lead to.

Diets don't work

We have in the last two generations become obsessed with dieting, but it's increasingly clear that faddish regimes and strict calorie counting don't work. Most people will have dipped their toe in and tried a diet at some point, but after an initial weight loss or burst of enthusiasm, the inevitable happens and the diet falls by the wayside. Despite doctors' advice over the last thirty years to eat less and exercise more, our waistlines are increasing, obesity is rising fast across the globe and weight-related diseases are more prevalent. But this is not simply a collective failure of willpower, as babies and infants have also been getting bigger. At the same time food allergy has become an epidemic and, despite the first modern case only being reported in 1969, it now affects nearly one in ten children. What research has shown is that our health, and in particular our weight, is governed by the key role of an until recently overlooked and outwardly invisible component: our microbiome.

The importance of our microbiome

Microbes describe any living creature that you need a powerful lens or microscope to see. We are surrounded by them in the air we breathe and the soil we garden with and play in; they are on our skin and in the food we eat. But we actually carry most of them around inside us in our intestines.

The four to five feet of the adult colon contains around 100 trillion microbes; these weigh as much as our liver and should be thought of as a newly discovered organ. Our microbes outnumber our own human cells ten to one (if you discount our borning non-replicating red blood cells) and have over 150 times more genes than we do.

We share about a third of our genes with our microbes, the original inhabitants of our planet from whom we slowly evolved millions of years ago. Since then we have provided them with a safe place to live plus a steady source of food. In return they have kept us healthy by controlling our immune systems, protecting us from invading aggressive microbes and helping us digest our food by extracting key chemicals and vitamins we require.

What do microbes do?

- Control our immune systems
- Protect us from invading aggressive microbes
- Help us digest food by extracting key chemicals and vitamins
- Produce chemicals altering our mood and appetite

The traditional view of microbes is based on stories of extreme food poisoning (such as salmonella), infections like pneumonia or potentially lethal diseases like gangrene. More recently so-called 'superbugs' (like MRSA or C. difficile) have hit the headlines because they have acquired resistance to antibiotics. By decimating the normal microbe community in the blood or bowel they dominate with fatal consequences. Yet these potentially 'bad' microbes make up less than 1 per cent of our microbiome (the combined set of our individual microbes) and usually exist in small numbers without harm to us.

Over the past fifty or so years we have been systematically destroying our microbiome by eating an increasingly processed and limited diet, becoming obsessed with cleanliness and hygiene and by the high instances of caesarean sections. Another major factor is antibiotic use which our ancestors and their microbes never experienced. Fewer than 1 in 500 people are spared antibiotics during their lifetime with the vast majority of adults in the UK and USA having an average of nearly one course for every year of life. Although they can be life-saving, most courses are unnecessary and regular courses of antibiotics can harm your microbiome permanently and increase your risk of obesity and allergy.

Did you know...

Regular courses of antibiotics can wipe out gut microbes and could make it harder for you to lose weight.

Sadly, antibiotics are widely used in farming and many meat products now contain small amounts of antibiotics which we end up ingesting. In short, we have been systematically decimating our microbiome and consequently increasing our susceptibility to illness, allergies and obesity by failing to embrace and care for this vital organ in our bodies.

Simply put, the greater the diversity of microbes you have, the healthier you are. Almost every study into common and chronic diseases has shown that people with poor gut health are at increased risk of illness and, moreover, are unable to fight back effectively against disease. The good news is, though, that you can improve your gut diversity and this is what these recipes are designed to help you do.

How to eat for a healthy microbiome

Our microbiome is crucial to our wellbeing and we need to feed it well. The processed food that is widely consumed, even if it purports to be 'healthy', is generally very low in crucial fibre which our microbes need in order to thrive and reproduce. Not only do processed foods lack fibre but they also contain chemicals which have a detrimental effect on our microbiome. For example, recent studies of emulsifiers (binding agents found commonly in sauces such as mayonnaise and ketchup as well as soya and meat products) have shown that they have the side effect of clumping together gut microbes, thus reducing their diversity and making them produce abnormal-fat producing chemicals. Another study looked at a range of common artificial sweeteners like aspartame, sucralose and saccharine and their effect on rodents and humans. Again, the results were very worrying. They all caused abnormal microbial profiles in humans with a loss of diversity and produced chemicals likely to increase the risk of diabetes. These studies show there is no such thing as a free lunch. By eating processed foods or going for zero-sugar or zero-fat products to reduce calories you will be adding many unwanted chemicals to your microbes' menu and making them less healthy. A similar pattern is emerging with pesticides in food.

The clear message by now is that you should say goodbye to processed foods. These include most ready meals which have many added chemicals designed to increase shelf life. What you need to be feeding your microbiome is a diverse diet high in fibre and rich in unprocessed vegetables, fruits, grains, unpasteurised cheeses and limited fish and meat, and you should aim to introduce as many new and different ingredients as possible. By eating a varied diet your gut will host a broader range of microbe species. This allows them to keep rogue microbes at bay, to recycle all your nutrients, and to have optimal numbers of genes and chemicals at your disposal to keep your immune system in balance.

How to eat for optimal health

Avoid processed foods and foods and drinks containing artificial sweeteners and eat a diverse diet high in fibre and rich in unprocessed vegetables, fruits, grains, unpasteurised cheeses, limited fish and meat, introducing as many new and different ingredients as possible.

The fruit and vegetables that you eat are made up of hundreds of different components and chemicals. Some provide the taste and others energy, which is released via glucose, whilst others still are not immediately beneficial to you but are crucial for your microbes. These are termed prebiotics. Just like the bits of wood that get broken down by microbes in your garden soil, so the hard-to-digest pieces of food (as in all mammals) can only be digested by enzymes secreted by your gut microbes. There are many hard-to-digest forms of fibre – the most well known is inulin. This is found in very high levels only in certain vegetables including chicory roots and Jerusalem artichokes, and in high levels in globe artichokes, leeks, celery, onions, garlic, asparagus and yams, as well as in lower levels in some fruits including bananas. Inulin is also found in wheat. Beans and other pulses are excellent sources of microbe-friendly fibre too.

The importance of fibre

With modern diet debates focusing on sugar and fat, we have ignored fibre. Most people in this country now eat less than half the amount of fibre needed to keep their microbes happy. Our microbes depend on undigested fibre reaching them in the colon to survive and reproduce. In return for fermenting our fibre and recycling our waste, our microbes liberate many key nutrients and a third of our vitamins and produce brain chemicals like serotonin which can alter our mood and appetite. They also produce chemicals called short-chain fatty acids (such as butyrate) which provide us with 6 per cent of our calories, but more importantly are key signallers to dampen down our immune system in the gut lining communicating with our blood. The more butyrate produced, the happier they (and you) are and the less likely you are to develop allergies or autoimmune diseases.

Our microbes also use as a fuel source chemicals called polyphenols which are released when certain foods are fermented in the colon. Polyphenols have been known generally as antioxidants for a while but their mechanism was, until recently, unclear. The list of healthy foods that have high polyphenol counts includes some surprises. As well as a range of brightly coloured fruit and vegetables such as apples, grapes, berries, red peppers and beans, there are lots of food types that have in the past been perceived as unhealthy. Recent large epidemiological studies have shown that not only are these foods not harmful, they offer protection from common diseases like heart disease and cancer. This previously 'naughty' but now nice list includes coffee beans, dark chocolate (70 per cent or more cocoa), peanuts and other nuts and seeds, olive oil (only if good-quality extra virgin) and – breathe a sigh of relief – wine (red being slightly better than white).

Load up on polyphenols

- Eat more brightly coloured vegetables and fruit.
- Enjoy drinking coffee and eating dark chocolate.
- Tuck into nuts and seeds.
- Use extra virgin olive oil.
- Drink red wine.

The benefits of eating more dairy

Other foods that our microbes embrace but that we have recently been told to avoid are dairy products high in saturated fats. While yogurt has always had a reasonable press, cheese high in fat has been much maligned because of spurious associations with cholesterol, despite the fact that the French eat twice as much as Anglo-Saxons do but have less heart disease.

Studies have shown that eating 'real' (unprocessed) cheese regularly is associated with a consistently lower risk of heart problems, while the evidence for milk and butter is less clear-cut. However, studies do indicate that milk may have protective properties while butter is certainly much better for heart health than artificial margarines.

The reason dairy products such as yogurt and cheese are healthy for most of us is that they are a form of probiotic. They are packed with microbes which feed off the lactose and produce lactic acid that keeps other potentially harmful microbes away. There are billions of bacteria and fungi in a crumb of cheese and many make it past your acidic stomach and settle briefly in your colon where they mingle happily with the long-term residents, improving their wellbeing and your metabolism.

Most microbes from dairy and probiotics are transient, meaning they don't hang around in your gut for long, and therefore need to be ingested regularly.

How fermented foods help

Fermented foods (foods produced by the action of microbes) work in a similar way to dairy and can have a range of bacteria and fungi. Kefir is a fermented milk that can contain hundreds of different microbes and there are many fermented soya-based foods used in Asian cooking like miso, natto, tempeh and tofu. Fermented cabbage (sauerkraut and kimchi) and pickles have been eaten for centuries and as well as being packed with microbes, they act as a combined pre- and probiotic as the cabbage fibre provides food for gut microbes. There is a whole range of fermented foods being rediscovered, including some like sourdough bread that you may not have thought about. Kombucha, fermented tea, is another that is becoming popular; it is made using a starter pack of a gooey blob of hundreds of different microbes including both lactic and acetic acid-producing bacteria and a variety of yeasts (see page 47). There is, of course, now a huge industry producing dietary supplements, including probiotics, but the diversity of bacteria found in commercial probiotic supplements is very limited. I favour embracing pre- and probiotics in synergy – eating foods that are high in pre- and probiotics together (banana or berries with yogurt, for example).

Diversity is the key

It's key to remember that our gut microbes can reproduce every thirty minutes and, given the right food and environment, can produce millions of generations in just a year of our lives. In order to show this at the extreme, my university student son Tom agreed to go on a fast food only diet for ten days. He could only eat burgers, chicken nuggets and soft drinks. After the ten days he had lost 40 per cent of his microbe species and felt lethargic and sick. Other such studies have shown very swift changes in the microbiome when adopting a diet that is concentrated on a narrow range of food types. The lack of fibre in most processed food (in Tom's case only found in the sliver of gherkin in the burger) is a major culprit but so too were the added chemicals that are now commonplace. With narrowed diets and diminished microbiomes, hygienic zeal and antibiotic overuse we are becoming more and more susceptible to disease, obesity and allergies. The good news is that armed with the latest scientific and medical knowledge, you can rebuild your gut microbe community.

So, as well as increasing the breadth of your daily diet, you may also want to try something else – namely intermittent fasting (best known as the 5:2 diet championed by Michael Mosley). Other than losing a few extra pounds, recent data suggests that microbes enjoy fasting and that this further kick-starts your gut microbiome into action, enhancing your beneficial microbes.

The recipes that Justine has created embrace diversity and, as well as being delicious, will boost your gut flora and help to ward off illness and improve your immune system. It's helpful to remember that with trillions of microbes inside you, you never have to eat alone. Hopefully with this knowledge and use of this book you will change your relationship with food for ever. Good luck.

Professor Tim Spector

Introduction

Over two years ago I read *The Diet Myth*, Professor Tim Spector's brilliant book on food, nutrition and microbes. I was so blown away by what I read that I was desperate to write a recipe book to partner his research. The research into good gut health is so new, and the field so lively and varied, that I've read hundreds of reports, articles, features and studies in order to understand just how clever our digestive systems are.

With such a lot of misinformation around, getting to the bottom of the subject (no pun intended) has been a time-consuming, occasionally frustrating but ultimately eye-opening experience. Who would have thought that the tiny organisms living within us could have such a massive impact on our health? There is still so much to learn, but scientists are making progress slowly but surely. Open-source academic studies like the American and British Gut Projects are helping enormously by studying the microbes of real people, by analysing their poo, to find out exactly which bacteria colonise our guts and how they could affect our health. Studies like MapMyGut commercial project are now aiming to personalise healthy diets based on your individual microbiomes (read more about this research on page 114.)

While scientists continue to make discoveries about the body's least glamorous but most fascinating organ, we should be guided by the strongest current findings. As Tim says, those point in no uncertain terms to a diverse diet rich in vegetables and fruit, beans, pulses and wholegrains, with some dairy, a moderate amount of poultry and fish and occasional red meat. Those ingredients are what the recipes in this book focus on.

This book

I'm not the only writer who's been excited by the possibilities of eating for good gut health. There are plenty of books out there, but I wanted to write this one, which is aimed mainly at people wanting to lose a few pounds while improving their overall health. You might not have loads of time on your hands, or unlimited funds for fancy ingredients. But, like me, you may want to boost your health as painlessly as possible. If you've read a bit about the importance of good gut health, and need a helping hand to discover more, you'll find it here. This is a book packed with recipes, tips and information and a simple meal plan that's easy to follow and useful enough to help anyone get on track with as little fuss as possible. There's no avoidance of food groups, no miracle cleanses, no week-long detoxes, just straightforward advice and a real-life approach to good, gut-healthy eating. If you have digestive issues, such as IBS, coeliac disease or other health problems to overcome, you will need specialised advice.

Writing this book involved trial, error and lots of onions, but the finished plan strikes a good balance.

My guiding principles were that it had to avoid:
- **strange ingredients**
- **lengthy preparation**
- **too much cooking**
- **dull and worthy dishes**

And it had to be:
- **gut-happy**
- **simple**
- **easy to follow**
- **flexible**
- **delicious!**

It's worked for me, so I'm pretty sure it will work for you too.

Eating well

To eat well, I need to plan ahead – but not so much that it interferes with my day-to-day life. I read somewhere about a method that involves cooking the whole week's vegetables on a Sunday, then putting them in jars to eat during the week. No thanks! I like my food to be freshly cooked (or frozen, then quickly reheated when the mood takes me). It not only tastes better, but it will contain a more plentiful supply of nutrients and it definitely doesn't need to be difficult or time-consuming. Luckily, for this plan diversity is the key. It's about eating different foods and treating your gut microbes to a variety of nutrients and fibre.

The plan

The 28-day plan is designed for two people but can easily be doubled up if you have a family to feed. On some days you will be cooking enough for four or six servings as I've created several dishes you can make ahead and freeze to save time later in the plan. In many ways, my recipes are pretty similar to what you might be cooking already. OK, there are probably a lot more vegetables than you are used to eating – and I'll be introducing extra beans and lentils. But there's nothing too scary, and you'll find the recipes so delicious that you'll want to cook them again and again. They don't call for any wacky ingredients, and only use stuff that you can buy in the supermarket. If you are under pressure and don't have time to cook, I've also given ideas for alternatives that you can buy from shops or eat in a restaurant.

You're likely to find that you're spending more on fresh fruit and vegetables, but a lot less on meat and chicken. That's because I want you to go meat-free three nights a week and as many lunchtimes as possible. I found that the easiest way to cut down on meat and chicken – and we were big meat-eaters in our family – was to make all Mondays, Wednesdays and Fridays meat-free. That made it a whole lot easier to plan weekly meals. My 28-day plan does the thinking for you, but try and stick to the principles when you're off-plan, because eating less meat is good for your health, especially your gut health.

Ideally, stick to the plan for 28 days to get the best of the balanced, nutritionally varied selection of recipes. If there is something you really don't fancy, though, swap it for something else you've already tried and liked or one of the other recipes in the book.

Eat just enough

We all eat far too much, and it's easily done. With an overriding fear of ever being hungry, so many of us overfeed ourselves. We suffer the consequences, with weight gain, heart disease, diabetes and cancer jostling for position at the top of the list.

The Mediterranean diet, which this plan is based on, was first identified as beneficial to health in the 1950s following studies in seven countries around the world. The communities that were living so well on the Mediterranean diet in Greece and Italy were mainly rural, and would not have enjoyed the abundance – or portion sizes – we do now. Food is so plentiful for most of us these days, we can eat a huge amount without really noticing. My plan is portion controlled – the recipes are designed to serve a certain number of people. Try not to be greedy and override the portion sizes. Get used to eating just enough, eating slowly and without distractions so that you notice when you're full. If your work is very physical or you exercise a lot, you may need to eat more – but try and stick to the good stuff and top up with extra vegetables and wholegrains rather than snacking.

You should find that by eating well, you will supply your body with all the nutrients it needs and any food cravings will diminish or disappear altogether (I've stopped craving great big hunks of cheddar, for instance). It sounds strange, but it really does make sense. If we fuel our bodies with what they need instead of highly processed, high-sugar, high-fat rubbish, our brains – often guided by our guts – won't be desperately driving us to consume more food to make up for the nutrient deficit. We will feel nourished and content. It sounds a bit new-agey but it's true.

One of the best ways to learn what your gut needs is to find out exactly how it works. I've explained the workings of the gut in the simplest way possible. If it makes sense to me, it should make sense to you too. So, read on and discover your gut.

Justine Pattison

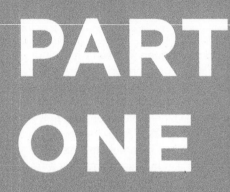

PART
ONE

1| What happens in the gut?

A brief introduction to your gut

Probably the easiest way to understand the workings of the gut is to imagine a long tube that travels from your mouth right through to your bottom. Food goes in at one end and is then digested by being broken down into smaller and smaller particles on its journey through your body. All the nutrients are absorbed, and what's left is excreted at the end as poo. Three-quarters of each poo is water, and the remaining waste consists of indigestible fibre, millions of dead and live bacteria, and a collection of other substances your body needs to get rid of (which could be cholesterol, food dye or the last bits of any medicine you've taken). Despite all the bacteria that exits your body in a poo, many trillions more are left happily colonising the gut.

An incredible journey

Imagine holding a crisp apple in your hand. Just looking at a soon-to-be snack will start your mouth watering, and your stomach will anticipate its arrival by producing digestive juices. Now imagine you're taking a big bite of the apple, forcing your teeth through the shiny skin and into the sweet, juicy flesh. Once it's in your mouth, your jaws bear down on their bite of apple, grinding and chewing, bursting the juice-filled cells and breaking it into smaller pieces ready for swallowing. As your jaws and tongue work together to round up the pieces of apple for their onward journey, your mouth continues to produce saliva. As well as keeping our mouths comfortable and helping us swallow, saliva does other, less obvious jobs. It helps protect our teeth, and the enzymes it contains start the digestion process.

Down the hatch

Once swallowed, the small pieces of apple mush, bound with saliva, travel down your oesophagus (also known as the gullet) and into your stomach. This stretchy, lopsided muscular pouch churns your food to break it down into small pieces. At the same time, the food is being combined with all sorts of enzymes and acids, known collectively as the gastric juices. These break down the food chemically even further. Only when most of the pieces are less than 2mm small are they ready to be welcomed by the small intestine.

What are enzymes?

Enzymes are proteins which act as enablers in our bodies, speeding up chemical reactions. They're involved in respiration as well as digestion, and outside the human body they're used in biological washing powder and food and drink manufacture. Some fruits contain an enzyme that breaks down gelatine, which is why you'll never see a kiwi or pineapple jelly.

Liquids travel relatively quickly through the curved, j-shaped stomach, while more solid foods are churned and mixed with gastric juices until broken up into tiny pieces and turned into a semi-liquid, partly digested mush called 'chyme'. Most absorption of nutrients takes place in the small intestine.

Did you know...?

Different foods spend differing amounts of time in the stomach. Like food scraps being pushed down the kitchen plughole by the lazy washer-upper, some are broken down and disappear into the next tube more readily than others. Simple carbs like white bread, rice or pasta are broken down relatively quickly, but it can be a few hours before protein-rich meat is ready for the small intestine. That's why steak keeps us feeling full for longer than pasta.

The small intestine

Our intestines' names refer to their width, rather than their length. The small intestine has a 2.5cm opening from the bottom of the stomach, but it has around six metres of coils and folds, like a long and untidy loop of butcher's sausages. Inside the tube and under a microscope, it actually looks more like a pink bathroom towel. The surface is made up of villi and microvilli, tiny fingers which maximise the surface area that comes into contact with our partly digested food.

with our partly digested food. As particles of our apple are squeezed, mixed and moved through the small intestine, nutrients are absorbed through its walls and into the bloodstream via tiny blood vessels in the villi. From here, the nutrient-rich blood goes to the liver, where any toxins are destroyed, and then onwards to wherever it might be needed. The last, tougher bits of food travel on to the large intestine.

Did you know...

An hour after the stomach and small intestine have finished digesting a piece of food, strong contractions sweep any remaining indigestible particles out of both areas and on into the large intestine. This cleaning process can only happen between meals. It's now thought to be crucial to efficient digestion, and could explain why frequent snacking with few breaks could have a detrimental effect on the body.

How useful is our appendix?

We might have put a man on the moon, but nobody knows exactly why we have an appendix. This small, thin pouch is connected to the large intestine, and has long been considered disposable. If you have appendicitis, your appendix will be removed. But research in the late noughties discovered that the healthy appendix is a warehouse for good bacteria. If a severe stomach upset strips the large intestine of friendly bacteria, the appendix supplies replacements.

The large intestine

By the time it leaves the small intestine, there isn't much left of our apple, just indigestible fibres, perhaps a seed or a bit of core swallowed as part of an enthusiastic bite. But there are still benefits to be had from the remnants, and this last bit of extraction happens in the large intestine.

Also known as the colon or bowel, the large intestine frames our small intestine on three sides. As well as hosting the absorption of the last remaining nutrients, it's also the home of our gut flora, or microbiome. The colon works at a much slower pace than the small intestine. By doing its job steadily, the large intestine has time to absorb minerals such as calcium and work with gut microbes to help convert food into fuel, make extra fatty acids and vitamins K, B12, B1 and B2. These help blood clot, strengthen the nervous system and are vital for a healthy brain and immune system.

The large intestine is also where water used in the digestion process is absorbed back into the body. The waste left behind solidifies into poo. If something disrupts the process (like anxiety or an infection), waste is released without any hanging around, resulting in loose, watery diarrhoea.

Your microbiome

The complex community of tiny microorganisms in your gut is called the microbiome. It contains hundreds of different types of microbes and these include bacteria, fungi and viruses. The great majority are bacteria. Most of the gut bacteria is found in the colon, or large intestine (bowel), the last part of the digestive tract where around 100 trillion bacteria are in residence.

The friendly gut bacteria perform many functions that are important for our health. They manufacture vitamins, including vitamin K and some B vitamins. They also turn fibre into short-chain fatty acids, which feed the gut wall and perform many other metabolic functions.

Obese people have different gut bacteria to lean people. Animal studies have shown that transplanting poo from lean mice can make fat mice lose weight. For this reason, many scientists now believe that our gut bacteria are important in determining our weight.

Because our overall health is governed to a surprising degree by these organisms, it's important to care for them. The study of gut microbes is in its infancy, but recent work has shown that diverse and abundant gut flora – which Tim advocates and my plan encourages – could have an impact on the following:

- **Obesity and our likelihood to gain weight**
- **Heart disease and high cholesterol**
- **Inflammatory diseases, especially those connected to the bowel**
- **Blood sugar control**
- **Brain function and mental health**
- **Immunity against disease**

Your microbiome

Microbes consist of bacteria, fungi, viruses and other types of tiny organisms.

The complex community of microorganisms in your gut is called the gut flora or gut microbiome (or microbiota).

The composition of gut flora can change over time and according to diet.

The balance of microbes in your gut depends on your diet. Certain microbes adapt according to what you eat, so someone who has a high-sugar diet is more likely to have a larger number of one bacteria, whereas a person who eats a lot of meat is more likely have a larger number of another. Scientists are just beginning to work out the impact that this balance has on our health.

It is believed that a diverse variety of microbes in your gut can hold the key to a range of health benefits.

• There are relatively few bacteria found in the stomach and small intestine, with the majority living in the large intestine (colon).

• Between 300 and 1,000 different species of bacteria can be found in the gut.

• Many species of bacteria from the gut cannot be studied outside the human body as they cannot be grown in laboratory conditions.

• There are a small number of core species that most of us carry but populations can vary widely between different people.

The bigger picture

Grasping the gut isn't always straightforward, especially as there's still so much research to be done. One of the easiest ways, I think, is to imagine you're in charge of a gorgeous garden and you want to encourage a variety of vigorous, healthy plants to grow there. The better the growing conditions, the bigger and stronger those plants will be, and the fewer aggressive weeds can break through and take over, depleting the soil and causing disease and decay. This is similar to looking after your internal microbial garden. You need to keep the good microbes flourishing so they'll outnumber any unwanted bacteria and viruses. You want to encourage them to multiply by feeding them all the foods they like best, a bit like giving a real garden fertiliser. Luckily, feeding a healthy gut means feeding yourself a rich variety of delicious food. What's more, it doesn't take long for the changes in your gut to start taking place, with gut microbes soon adjusting to the new diet while you reap the benefits.

Three steps to a healthy microbiome

For a healthy microbiome, you'll be eating more fermentable fibre and polyphenol-rich foods, supplemented by a regular intake of probiotics.

1 Fermentable fibre comes from plant sources, such as beans, lentils, onions, leeks and oats, and reaches the large intestine (colon) without being digested on its journey. Our microbes need this type of fibre in order to thrive and reproduce.

2 Some other foods, such as olive oil, red wine and chocolate, contain important chemicals called polyphenols which are released when fermented by gut bacteria.

3 Probiotic foods, such as live yogurt, are teeming with good bacteria that can support the existing bacteria in the gut and help prevent harmful bacteria taking over. It's a bit like having a peace-keeping force on board.

2| Eating for a healthy gut

The importance of fibre

We've all got a good gut feeling about fibre. But what is it, and why is it so useful to have around?

Fibre is a form of carbohydrate that humans can't digest, and can only be found in food that comes from plants. Traditionally, fibre is divided into two types, known as insoluble and soluble. We need both and, conveniently, nature often provides them together. The skin of an apple, for example, is rich in insoluble fibre, while its flesh is a good source of the soluble variety.

Fibre mostly passes through the digestive system unabsorbed because we don't have the enzymes needed to break it down. Nevertheless, its presence has a big effect on our health.

Soluble fibre

- Soluble fibre dissolves in the water in your gut to form a gel-like substance. It can reduce blood sugar spikes and has various health benefits including, researchers think, the reduction of blood cholesterol.

- Soluble fibre contains compounds called prebiotics, which act like microbe fertilizers and fuel the good bacteria in our gut. With the fuel to thrive, these friendly bacteria can dominate the bad ones, produce vitamins and aid the immune system.

- Research on prebiotics is ongoing at a feverish pace, but good sources we know about include leeks, onions, garlic, asparagus, legumes and artichokes.

Fermentable fibre

Fermentation is a healthy gut buzzword. Because both soluble and insoluble fibre can be fermented by friendly bacteria to produce good stuff, some researchers are abandoning the traditional 'does it dissolve?' question and asking 'does it ferment?' instead. But the soluble and insoluble categories are still a useful way to think about fibre, especially since most fermentable fibres are soluble.

Insoluble fibre

Insoluble fibre does not dissolve in water and passes through the digestive system mainly intact – think about that undigested corn kernel that you might have noticed in your poo. It functions mostly as a bulking agent and may help speed the passage of food and waste through your gut. It's found in wholemeal bread, bran, cereals, fibrous vegetables, nuts and seeds.

Resistant starch

A useful prebiotic, resistant starch is so-called because – surprise! – it's resistant to digestion. It passes through the digestive system unchanged, but good bacteria love it and will ferment it in a similar way to soluble fibre. It can be found in food such as green bananas, uncooked oats, cashew nuts, beans and lentils. Cooling some carbohydrate-rich foods after cooking also helps form resistant starch. As it cools, the starch crystallises and becomes more resistant to digestion, giving sushi rice and potato salad an edge over hotter stuff like stir-fried rice and roasties. Studies have also shown that eating resistant starch helps you feel fuller for longer; insoluble fibre has the same effect.

A word of warning

If you aren't used to eating much fibre in the form of wholegrains, beans and lentils particularly, or have existing digestive issues, it's best to start off a new fibre-rich eating regime slowly. You need to give the microbes in your gut time to get used to the new diet. Those specifically adapted to ferment various types of fibre will need to multiply and flourish, so they can handle the changes. If you don't take it easy to begin with, you could experience discomfort from excess bloating and wind.

The low FODMAP diet

Doctors and dietary specialists sometimes place patients with irritable bowel syndrome on what's known as a low FODMAP diet. FODMAP stands for fermentable oligosaccharides, disaccharides, monosaccharides and polyols. Avoiding these can produce good results in some patients, but means adopting a seriously restrictive regime. Wheat, legumes, pulses and some fruit and vegetables are all out – with an accompanying loss of fibre, nutrients, polyphenols and prebiotics. The health and diversity of the microbiome can suffer as a consequence.

Low FODMAP diets are not to be toyed with, and should be overseen by an expert dietician with the aim of slowly reintroducing foods to work out what the patient can and can't tolerate. While low FODMAP diets are helpful for only some IBS sufferers, this plan is almost the opposite of the low FODMAP diet, and should benefit most people, including those who haven't been helped by FODMAP diets. If you have any concerns about your digestion, you should see a doctor before you start this plan.

Prebiotics

Prebiotics and probiotics are different, but they are both forces for good in the gut. While probiotic foods contain good bacteria, prebiotics feed good bacteria. As we saw in the chapter on fibre, prebiotics are the parts of our food which fuel the good bacteria in the gut. They're found in non-digestible fibres, mainly from sources of soluble fibre including vegetables and fruit. Harmful bacteria can't make much use of prebiotics, but good bacteria thrive on them. When good bacteria grow in strength and number, they take the balance of power in the gut, and are able to do their excellent work unhindered while we stay fit and well.

In another example of excellent natural design, breast milk is a source of prebiotics. Understandably, lots of work has been done on isolating the particular compound (known as an oligosaccharide) which feeds infants' good bacteria – so breast milk research feeds our understanding of the microbiome, too. Inulin is another of science's prebiotic favourites and occurs in foods such as Jerusalem artichokes, leeks, onions and garlic.

Two 'flower' families of vegetables provide sources of many recognised prebiotics. Endives, chicory and Jerusalem artichokes are part of the sunflower family, while leeks and asparagus are both related to lilies.

- **Probiotics are selected microbes that have been shown to be good for us when we consume them, either as food or in supplements.**

- **Prebiotics are the elements of our food, found mainly in soluble fibre, which feed and fertilise good bacteria in the gut.**

Although all prebiotics are fibre, not all fibre is prebiotic. Prebiotic foods are high in special types of fermentable fibre that support digestive health by feeding the friendly bacteria in the gut. By promoting the increase of friendly bacteria in the gut, they help with digestive problems and even boost your immune system. Recent research even suggests that prebiotic fibre can help you sleep better and reduce stress due to the effect that happy gut microbes have on the brain.

My top ten prebiotics

If you want to keep your gut bacteria healthy and well fed, introduce more prebiotic fibre to your diet. All plant-based foods, such as fruit, vegetables and grains, contain fibre, but some are richer sources of fermentable prebiotic fibre than others. Here are my top ten:

- Garlic
- Onions
- Leeks
- Jerusalem artichokes
- Globe artichokes
- Asparagus
- Bananas
- Apples
- Wholegrain oats, wheat and barley
- Lentils and beans

GARLIC

As well as being an excellent source of polyphenols and vitamins, garlic is a first-class prebiotic.

How to buy and store

Check your garlic is nice and fresh, with dry papery skins; it shouldn't smell mouldy or have green shoots growing inside each clove. Keep in a bowl in the kitchen at room temperature, so it is always on hand. You can also freeze crushed garlic cloves in a small container and then spoon out and use from frozen. A teaspoon of frozen garlic is about the same as one large clove.

How to eat more

- It's worth doubling or tripling the amount of garlic you normally use for pasta sauces, stews and curries.
- Always add garlic raw to dressings or dips.
- Try roasting garlic whole to serve squeezed out of the skins. Slow-roasted garlic doesn't taste or smell nearly as pungent as raw garlic.

ONIONS

Onions are plentiful and cheap. I tend to choose the red ones because, as well as the prebiotic fibre that your microbes will love, the red colour indicates a particularly good source of antioxidants. Look out for shallots too as they have similar properties.

How to buy and store

Look for onions that are firm and dry. The papery skin should be fairly brittle and look shiny. Squidgy, damp onions could be mouldy inside. Keep in a cool place and don't buy too many at a time unless you are preparing them within a few days. I tend to keep mine in the fridge as my kitchen is warm and I don't want them to sprout – but I make sure they are in the salad drawer and away from any moisture.

How to eat more

• Onions are used in such a massive variety of recipes that it should be no problem incorporating them into your diet. Think about increasing the size of the onions you use or adding an extra half an onion to a dish occasionally.
• Spring onions and red onion also taste good raw, so slice finely and add to salads or use for salsas and relishes.
• Raw onion contains more fermentable fibre than cooked onion.
• If you don't like chopping onions, buy ready-chopped and frozen onions – or do it yourself in bulk.
• The key to hassle-free onions is to treat yourself to a decent knife; a nice sharp knife will make short work of the job.

Another great prebiotic vegetable that's quite cheap and easy to incorporate into other dishes. Leeks are also a great source of antioxidants, such as the flavonoid kaempferol, which is thought to help reduce the risk of developing chronic diseases and protect our blood vessels.

How to buy and store

Look for firm leeks with tight leaves. Trim off the root end 5mm in and remove any tough outer leaves from larger leeks. Trim the leaves down the length of the leek to the point the knife slides easily through. Supermarkets tend to sell them very well trimmed but they are more expensive bought that way.

How to eat more

- Leeks are generally considered a winter vegetable, but it is now possible to buy them all year round and you might also find baby leeks in early spring.
- Leeks can be used like onions and gently sautéed at the beginning of a recipe. Try cooking a sliced leek as well as the usual onion in any of your favourite recipes, such as bolognese, stews or risotto, for added prebiotic fibre.
- Leeks also make a great vegetable side dish – I add them to the same pan as other vegetables, such as carrots or beans, when I'm cooking, but just for the last 3–5 minutes of the cooking time.
- Leeks can also be stir-fried and tossed through cooked rice or potatoes and even boiled until soft, cooled and drizzled with vinaigrette as a light summer lunch.

JERUSALEM ARTICHOKES

Artichokes are a fantastic source of inulin, the special fermentable fibre that your gut microbes adore. The big dose of inulin they provide can disrupt your gut in a rather obvious manner, which is why Jerusalem artichokes are sometimes known as 'fartichokes'. Go easy with the portion size to begin with.

How to buy and store

A Jerusalem artichoke is a hard, knobbly tuber that looks a bit like a cross between a new potato and fresh root ginger. They are harvested between October and March, making them a delicious winter vegetable to add to your menu. Unfortunately, Jerusalem artichokes are difficult to find in supermarkets, but often appear in street markets and greengrocers at the right time of year. If you see some, grab them, or find out whether your greengrocer can order some for you. The flavour is very distinctive, being both sweet and slightly smoky. They remind me of roasted parsnip mashed with the flesh of a baked potato. Store Jerusalem artichokes in the fridge and try to eat them within a few days. They will keep for weeks, but are better eaten close to when they are harvested.

How to eat more

- Look for the artichokes with the fewest knobbles as they will be easier to peel. You can also cook them in their skins, but you need to make sure you brush really well between all the lumps and bumps to remove the soil.
- My favourite use for them is a silky Jerusalem artichoke soup, but you can also make a delicious purée to serve with grilled meats and fish or roasted vegetables.
- Blanch sliced artichokes in boiling water and then fry in a little olive oil until golden to use in a warm salad or even as a soup garnish.
- Jerusalem artichoke soup and purée freeze well, so it's worth making a big batch of both when they're in season.

Globe artichokes are the buds of a large member of the thistle family and are a useful source of inulin. You can eat the heart and the tender flesh at the bottom of the cooked leaves. Because artichokes are seasonal and a bit of a fiddle, I tend to buy the chargrilled artichoke hearts sold as antipasti.

How to buy and store

Artichokes have leaves growing tightly around a central heart and are simple, but rather time-consuming to prepare. Tiny artichokes can be eaten raw but you are unlikely to find them in the UK, so if you'd like to try fresh ones go for the larger, more mature kind. Look for firm, tightly packed green artichokes (they may have a purple blush) that feel heavy. Buy between June and the end of October, when they are at their best, and store in the fridge.

How to eat more

- The bottom part of each leaf and the heart of the bud are edible but the outer leaves and central furry 'choke' aren't.
- You can boil artichokes whole, with a little lemon juice added to the water to prevent them discolouring, and serve with a good garlicky vinaigrette.
- For a hands-on starter, take each leaf, dip into the vinaigrette and scrape off the fleshy part at the base with your teeth.
- You can also prepare artichokes right down to the hearts before boiling or roasting.
- Use ready-prepared artichoke hearts as part of your gut-happy lunch platter, or toss through salads, use as a topping for pizzas and blitz into dips.

ASPARAGUS

Asparagus is quick to prepare and cook and contains a useful proportion of inulin. It's a seasonal ingredient, and British asparagus is prized for its delicate flavour, but it is imported all year around.

How to buy and store

Look for firm stalks with a slightly glossy green colour and closed tips. Smaller stems are not always more tender – larger stalks have a better ratio of flesh to skin. Try to eat on the day you buy them, or trim the ends and store upright in a mug with a little cold water. Keep cool in the fridge and eat within a couple of days.

How to eat more

• Asparagus needs boiling for just 2–6 minutes, depending on its thickness, and can also be served raw, shaved or very thinly sliced, in salads.
• Try using asparagus as well as green beans, carrots or broccoli as an accompaniment to other dishes or add halved asparagus to risottos, omelettes and pasta dishes.
• For a symbiotic prebiotic and probiotic boost, try making a cooling soup with puréed asparagus cooked in stock, topped with live yogurt and fresh herbs.
• Simply cooked asparagus can also be served cold as part of a deli-style platter or for a packed lunch with a small pot of thick vinaigrette for dipping.

BANANAS

Greenish, underripe bananas contain more fermentable fibre than softer, yellow bananas. This is because they contain a particular kind of resistant starch which feeds beneficial bacteria in your gut. They ferment more slowly than other high-fibre foods, such as beans, Jerusalem artichokes and onions, so they're less likely to cause wind.

How to buy and store

Unripe bananas are pretty horrible to eat, so it's best to select those that are just beginning to ripen; they'll be pale greeny-yellow rather than pure green and will still contain lots of fibre. Most supermarkets sell underripe bananas ready for ripening at home. Just buy a few at a time and keep them in the fridge. The skins may start to darken but the banana shouldn't ripen any further.

How to eat more

• Sliced thinly, just-ripe bananas are perfect served on top of oats or on wholewheat pancakes for breakfast. You can get some probiotic–prebiotic symbiosis going by adding live yogurt.
• Bananas can also be tossed through salads or coarsely grated and served on top of spicy curries and chillies with yogurt as a gut-healthy relish.

APPLES

Research into frequent apple consumption has linked it to reduced risk of heart disease, some cancers, diabetes and weight loss. They are a rich source of polyphenols and a special fibre called pectin, as well as other soluble fibres, which reach the large intestine intact and can have a beneficial effect on gut microbes.

How to buy and store

Look for firm apples with no signs of damage or bruising. Buy frequently, use quickly and keep at room temperature. Try different varieties, focusing on old-fashioned, more acidic apples which will contain more pectin than the new varieties bred for sweetness. And don't forget about using cooking apples, such as Bramley, which are the richest in pectin.

How to eat more

- Eating at least one apple most days shouldn't be too difficult. They can be grated into oats and yogurt for a gut-healthy overnight muesli or stirred into porridge for breakfast.
- Toss them into salads for lunch or slice thinly and pile onto open proper cheese sandwiches.
- Sliced apple can be stir-fried or simmered in sauces.
- Cooking apples can be stewed with dried fruits for sweetness and a little cinnamon for pudding or to serve cold with yogurt for breakfast.
- Try using as a filling for pies or serve as relish with cooked meats, especially pork, or unpasteurised cheeses.

Oats and barley are high in a type of fermentable soluble fibre called beta-glucans, which can help lower blood cholesterol and reduce the risk of diabetes. Wheat contains types of soluble fibre that have been found to increase beneficial bacteria in the gut, boosting the immune system and helping to reduce blood sugar levels.

How to buy and store

Porridge oats, pearl barley and wholemeal bread and pasta are easy to buy and can be stored at room temperature. Buy porridge oats that are minimally processed, such as jumbo oats, rather than tubs of instant oats with added sugar. You can also buy oats with added wheat bran for extra fibre. Pearl barley has had varying amounts of its bran 'polished' away and isn't as high in fibre as the unpolished version, but it still contains good amounts of soluble fibre and is easier to get hold of. Buy or make wholemeal bread (see my note about bread and additives on page 136) and choose wholewheat pasta and noodles.

How to eat more

- Eat oats for breakfast, as muesli, porridge or granola. At least three days a week is good, but more is even better.
- You can also use oats for crumble toppings and whizzed to a powder for pancakes and coatings for fried fish.
- Pearl barley can be simmered in stews, made into healthy risottos and cooked and cooled for gut-happy salads.
- Wholegrain wheat kernels are sometimes known as wheat berries and look similar to pearl barley. They have a delicious, slightly sweet, nutty flavour but take around an hour to soften in boiling water. Soaking them overnight will help them cook more quickly.
- Use stoneground wholemeal flour for baking, swapping for roughly half of the white flour in your usual recipes. It will soak up more liquid, so be prepared to adjust the quantities accordingly.

LENTILS AND BEANS

The term 'legume' refers to plants whose fruit is enclosed in a pod, such as peas and beans. Pulses are part of the legume family, but the term 'pulse' refers to only the dried seeds. Pulses include dried beans and lentils. They are a cheap source of protein, fibre, vitamins and minerals. Pulses are low in fat and packed with soluble fibre that gut microbes love to use for energy. This helps lower cholesterol and keeps blood sugar levels stable. Some people are put off eating beans because the fermentation of the soluble fibre can cause flatulence. But if you avoid these hard-to-digest carbohydrates, your gut microbes will be missing out. Instead, start off slowly and gradually build up the amount you eat each week. That way, your internal flora will have a chance to adapt better and windy symptoms should be reduced.

How to buy and store

Pulses are usually sold in bags ready for cooking at home, or can be bought cooked in cans, cartons and jars. Foods like hummus are made from pulses that have been blended to form a dip, and you can get chickpea (or 'gram') flour which can be added to flatbreads. Other common pulses include baked beans and the red kidney beans that you might use for a chilli con carne.

How to eat more

- Easy-to-find pulses include red, green, yellow and brown lentils, chickpeas, black-eyed peas, kidney beans, butter beans, haricot beans, cannellini beans, flageolet beans, pinto beans and borlotti beans.
- Stir into soups and stews, simmer in curries and toss with salads.
- You can use mashed lentils and beans for gut-happy dips and spread on hot toast too.
- Try swapping a proportion of the meat in a casserole or curry for pulses, increasing the amount each time. You'll be adding useful fibre and making the dish much cheaper to boot.
- Cook big batches of dried beans and store in the freezer to reheat quickly from frozen.

Fermentable fibre

I think gut health is a fascinating subject – and most of the internet agrees with me. Online searches may suggest some sources of fermentable fibre which are hard to find. Here's my take…

Chicory root is a fantastic source of inulin (fermentable fibre) but it is almost impossible to buy. You may find dried chicory powders and chicory root 'coffee' in health food shops, but with a large selection of other inulin-rich foods available, it's not top of my shopping list. As a salad vegetable, chicory is great for variety but doesn't have the same properties as the root.

The same goes for dandelion root, burdock and any of the other roots you might see on prebiotic lists. They're fabulous sources of inulin, but at the moment, they are very difficult to get hold of – I'd rather spend that time cooking, eating and enjoying other foods. Maybe in the future, as gut health becomes more mainstream, all these roots will be readily available in the supermarket and no more difficult to buy than a bag of potatoes.

Did you know…

- Research has shown that introducing more fibre to the gut can reduce the number of microbes associated with weight gain and increase those linked to leanness.
- Studies have revealed that when microbes are starved of fibre they can start to feed off the protective mucus lining of the gut, possibly causing inflammation and disease.
- One particular strain of bacteria associated with weight loss needs the mucus in the gut to survive and flourish.

Probiotics

In modern times, we've been convinced that all bacteria are bad. Many of us rush around sanitising everything and trying to get rid of '99% of all germs', or whatever the label on a cleaning product promises us. We flood our bodies with antibiotics to kill these germs but at the same time wipe out the good microbes that live in and alongside us and are now known to provide numerous health benefits.

Probiotics are live microorganisms (microbes), usually bacteria, that when eaten in adequate amounts, provide a health benefit for the host (that's us). Probiotics crop up naturally in lots of foods, such as traditionally made yogurt and cheese and fermented pickles. You're also bound to have seen little yogurt drinks with added probiotic bacteria crowding the chiller department of your local supermarket. They're expensive and often oversweetened, and I'm not convinced about their effectiveness. There's also no guarantee that the particular strains of bacteria they contain will suit me, so I'd rather aim for variety and try a range of good yogurt and cheese.

Probiotics help balance our microbiome and stimulate the digestive system to take tiny but valuable steps to protect our bodies from harm. They're essential for a healthy gut, and their role is particularly important when our systems are under pressure from antibiotics.

Eating and drinking probiotics can feel like a leap of faith, and there's still a lot to discover about how they work. As we know, though, it's a long, tough journey to the large intestine, and it's believed that the bacteria in probiotics need to make it there alive in order to do the most good. The ones that do get there don't usually hang around for long – but they have an impact on the gut microbiota nonetheless.

There are dozens of probiotic bacteria that have been shown to have health benefits. The most common groups include lactobacillus and bifidobacterium, names you may have seen on the label of your favourite yogurt.

There are many different species within each group and each

species has many different strains. For most benefits, it's worth eating lots of different probiotic foods, so you treat your gut to plenty of microbiological variety. Yogurt and unpasteurised raw milk cheeses are relatively easy to get hold of but there are other probiotics, such as kefir and kimchi, which are growing in popularity.

There's no need to go mad with probiotics. Just eat at least one serving of a probiotic food with each meal if you can. Simply having live natural yogurt for breakfast or adding a few spoonfuls on top of a curry or chilli with your evening meal will help to begin with. Then you can start introducing some of the other probiotics. They can be bought, but it's also interesting, and quite good fun, to make your own. Make sure that any 'starter' products, such as kombucha SCOBYs or kefir grains are bought from a reputable supplier.

My top five probiotics

- **Natural live yogurt**
- **Unpasteurised cheese**
- **Kimchi**
- **Kefir**
- **Kombucha**

NATURAL LIVE YOGURT

Live yogurt gets its sharp flavour from the acid produced during fermentation. It's one of the easiest probiotics to recommend because there's decent evidence that eating it can benefit health. The lactobacilli and bifidobacteria in yogurt have even been shown to affect centres in the brain, and some research demonstrates that the consumption of yogurt microbes alters the way we break down other foods – for the better.

If microbes are listed on your yogurt label, look for a count of over five billion CFUs (colony-forming units) to ensure there's enough in each spoonful to reach your large intestine. Full-fat yogurt tastes better with its rich, round flavour. Greek yogurt is fine too, as long as it contains live bacteria. Avoid sweetened versions, or those with fruit flavours – your own fruit toppings will have more fibre and polyphenols.

How to eat more

- Eat simply for breakfast, topped with berries, nuts and seeds.
- Whizz up with fresh fruit and chill in the fridge to make your own sugar-free probiotic shot drink.
- Mix with crushed garlic and herbs, or leftover soft cheese, for a tangy yogurt dip to serve with vegetable sticks as a light meal.
- Make into dressings by adding herbs, spices and extra virgin olive oil or mixing with blue cheese.
- Blend juicy berries with live yogurt to make your own sugar-free desserts or stir in a few rolled oats and slacken with milk for a filling smoothie with a probiotic boost.
- Make your own 'yogurt cheese' (labneh), see my recipe on page 246. Making your own soft cheese with full-fat live yogurt should guarantee that it's teaming with beneficial bacteria. Serve spread onto toast, mix with garlic and herbs for lunch or scoop onto softly poached fruits.

Made with milk that hasn't been heat-treated to kill off microorganisms, unpasteurised or raw milk cheese has the potential to be a probiotic feast for the gut. There's a theory that the extra microbes in traditional cheeses (not processed) could prevent some heart and other health problems. Even cheese made with pasteurised milk will contain plenty of microbes as the cheese is fermented with bacteria after heat treating, just not the diversity found in raw milk cheeses.

Mould-ripened cheeses, such as brie and camembert, and soft, blue-veined cheeses, such as gorgonzola and Roquefort, are less acidic than hard cheeses and contain more moisture. They provide the perfect environment for all sorts of bacteria to grow.

Eat a small amount of a range of unpasteurised raw milk cheeses, maybe three to four at most, rather than a lot of just one variety. Don't buy the same ones each week – chop and change a bit.

How to eat more

- Check out your local deli or cheese shop, if you have one. Ask about unpasteurised/raw milk cheeses and buy thin slices to try.
- If using cheese in hot food, add at the end of the cooking time, so the heat doesn't destroy all those beneficial bacteria.
- Eat like a Northern European. Try having small slices or chunks of cheese for breakfast and serve with hard-boiled eggs, maybe a slice of organic ham and wholegrain bread.

A word of warning

Certain groups should avoid eating soft, mould-ripened or blue cheeses made from unpasteurised milk as they are more at risk of illness when harmful bacteria, such as listeria, are consumed in foods. These include very young children, the elderly, pregnant women and those whose immune system is compromised.

KIMCHI

Traditionally made in almost every Korean home, this spicy cabbage relish is the national dish. It's now widely known outside its home country for its digestive benefits and the kick and crunch it can add to all kinds of dishes.

Traditional kimchi is fermented, with a long shelf life thanks to the lactic acid produced during the process. If you're buying it, look for a jar that hasn't been heat-treated, which would destroy its probiotic properties. If you don't like things spicy, you could try sauerkraut or other fermented pickled vegetables instead. Sauerkraut and fermented pickled vegetables are incredibly easy to prepare and simply require dunking in a light salt solution. Before long, the lactic acid bacteria begin the fermentation process and effectively preserves the vegetables.

There are some brilliant fermentation books available with detailed instructions on how to prepare your veg, so I haven't given any specific recipes here. Once you get used to this new way of eating, it's good to experiment with new foods and fermented vegetables contain a brilliant combination of probiotic and prebiotic properties.

How to eat more

- Serve alongside Asian-style stir fries and noodle dishes.
- Mix into egg-fried rice after it comes off the hob – you don't want the heat to kill any of the beneficial bacteria.
- Spoon kimchi over toast and top with grated cheese then flash under the grill.
- Use as a filling for omelettes, or even stir into scrambled eggs if you are feeling brave, adding at the end of the cooking time.
- Stir through potato salad made with crème fraiche and yogurt for a spice-filled fix.
- Use as a topping for burgers, or as a tangy salsa for barbecued or roasted meats.

A slightly sharp cultured drink made mainly with milk, kefir contains lots of different strains of bacteria and beneficial yeast and is a wonderful source of probiotics. It's also rich in B and K vitamins. It was traditionally fermented in the Caucasus mountains but word has spread and it can now be bought ready-made, although it is easy to make at home using a starter of kefir 'grains' and the milk of your choice. Kefir is a bit of an acquired taste and I didn't enjoy the kefir I made during research for this book as it was incredibly sour. I've since learnt that an easy way to get milk kefir into your diet is to eat muesli with half yogurt and half kefir, lots of cinnamon and a drizzle of honey. Different methods of fermentation will also give different degrees of sourness. Coconut kefir is now widely available too.

You could also try water kefir, which is made with grains which metabolise the sugars in sweetened water to make a gently fizzy probiotic tonic. I have read that our love of fizzy drinks harks back to the days when fermented kefir-like liquids were an important part of our diets and there is definitely something appealing about home made water kefir. I've also made a delicious ginger beer at home using a specific 'starter', but the huge quantity of sugar it required would have drastically reduced any benefits.

It's very easy to buy kefir grains online and they come with detailed instructions on how to make the drinks. Like anything that's live, kefir needs looking after to make sure it is fed with the right sugars and stored correctly so the bacteria can do their job – it's quite a responsibility but it's also exciting tasting the results.

How to eat more

- Mix milk kefir into live yogurt to give an extra probiotic boost, and serve with fresh berries or lightly poached fruit.
- Stir milk kefir into dips and dressings to add lots of beneficial bacteria.
- Add water kefir to assorted chopped fruit and serve as a fruit salad, topped with crème fraiche or live yogurt.
- Prepare shots of milk or water kefir in small glass jars or bottles and get in the habit of drinking once a day.

KOMBUCHA

This fizzy, fermented tea originated in China and has been enthusiastically adopted in Japan, Russia and Eastern Europe. It's now popular in the West, too, but commercially available versions can contain a lot of sugar, and it's easy to make at home. Tea is fermented with what's known as a symbiotic culture of bacteria and yeast, or a SCOBY, which looks a bit like a yellowy-brown disc of jelly.

A variety of outlandish health claims have been made for kombucha, but I think of it simply as a useful probiotic which is rich in gut-happy bacteria. It tastes like a slightly fizzy apple juice and is very simple to make at home. After the surprise of the first sip, it doesn't take long to get used to the tangy flavour. You can buy a live SCOBY online and then add it to a jar of sweetened black tea. After a few days fermentation, the kombucha is ready to drink. And you use the same SCOBY to make the next batch. Again, the instructions that come with the SCOBYs that I've bought online have been very detailed, so there's not much to go wrong. I found the biggest problem with fermenting my own kombucha was storing the massive jar it was made in and finding space in the fridge for the subsequent bottles of kombucha.

How to eat more

- Give iced tea a probiotic advantage by mixing with home-made kombucha.
- Stir kombucha into dressings and drizzle over salad.
- Mix with water, fresh mint and sliced lemon for a refreshing post work-out drink.

Other gut-friendly foods

Think your gut microbes only thrive on goody-two-shoes foods? Not so. Surprisingly, your microbiome savours some of life's little luxuries just as much as you do. The benefits mainly seem to be due to the polyphenols these foods contain, sometimes with a good boost of fibre too. Here's a brief guide to what they are and how to enjoy them.

What are polyphenols?

Polyphenols are natural compounds found in certain foods, including fruit and vegetables, which have special properties. They're the subject of continuing research and are believed to have a positive effect on our risk of developing heart disease, diabetes, cancer and dementia. But polyphenols also seem to actively encourage some microbes to flourish. These include microbes such as the lactobacilli that mop up and bind fatty particles, and clear them from the blood. Theses beneficial microbes also prevent unwanted microbes from colonising our guts. This reduces the incidence of infection from bugs that can cause diarrhoea, stomach ulcers, pneumonia and even tooth decay.

Five surprisingly gut-friendly foods

- Olive oil
- Nuts
- Chocolate
- Red wine
- Coffee

OLIVE OIL

Good-quality extra virgin olive oil contains the greatest amounts of polyphenols. It's produced with the very minimum of processing, so it retains the best flavour and nutrients. Virgin oil is NOT as good, and oils described as 'light' or 'simply olive oil' are best avoided as they have been chemically refined, and lack the antioxidants and anti-inflammatories found in extra virgin olive oil. They tend to be used in olive oil spreads and oils designed for cooking.

When we eat extra virgin olive oil, over 80 per cent of its fatty acids and nutrients make it to the colon before full digestion has taken place. This allows our microbes to feast on these polyphenols and fatty acids, breaking them down into even smaller and very useful compounds. These signal to the body to lower harmful lipid levels, while good bacteria are supported and bad ones are prevented from taking over.

The Mediterranean diet is one of the most researched in the world. All the indications are that extra virgin olive oil and nuts, eaten alongside the basic Mediterranean provisions of vegetables, grains and pulses, reduce the incidence of disease and early death. The Mediterranean diet is also associated with maintaining a healthy weight.

How to buy and store

Light is the enemy of good olive oil, so buy it in a dark glass bottle and store it in a cool, dark place – resist keeping it next to the hob. Buy the best quality that you can afford, and check that your bottle has a long best-before date (some even display the date of harvest) so you know it's as fresh as possible. And don't forget that olives are also good for you, so add them to as many dishes as possible. Green olives have more polyphenols than black ones. Some olives are more natural than others – black olives which have been pitted and look very black may have been treated with chemicals to colour them, so choose those with a purple, dark grey or browny-black colour – Kalamata are usually a good bet.

How to eat more

- Use extra virgin olive oil rather than sunflower or vegetable oil or butter most of the time.
- Use for dipping bread instead of serving it with butter – add a little balsamic vinegar if you like.
- Whisk into dressings to serve on salads (see recipes on pages 292–295). Serving leafy salads with an olive oil dressing actually makes the vitamins more available for your body to use.
- Use olive oil in marinades for meat, chicken and fish. It's great for imparting flavour and keeping the meat succulent as it cooks.
- Drizzle olive oil over fresh vegetable chunks, season and sprinkle with herbs and roast until tender.
- Try making your own pesto with nuts, olive oil, fresh basil, garlic and Grana Padano (an unpasteurised hard cheese similar to Parmesan) – a huge amount of gut-friendly ingredients all in one! (See recipe on page 155.)
- Serve a bowl of olives instead of highly processed crisps or similar snacks. Toss olives into salads and stir into pasta sauces and casseroles.
- Make a rich olive tapenade spread for smearing onto fresh bread or toast by blending olives with garlic and olive oil, plus capers and anchovies.

NUTS

Nuts are good sources of healthy fats, protein, fibre, vitamins and minerals, but they also contain useful polyphenols. Walnuts contain the most antioxidant polyphenols, with Brazil nuts and pistachios also near the top of the list. Studies have shown that roasting nuts helps boost the available level of polyphenols, too.

No one would deny that they're very high in calories, but it has been shown that eating nuts as a morning snack can help prevent overeating later in the day. It's not clear exactly why, but one theory is that it's connected to the gut. Importantly, it's also recently been shown that the calorie content of nuts has been overestimated by up to 20 per cent.

As you may have noticed, when you eat whole nuts not all of the nut is broken down and absorbed by the body. This means that not all the calories have been available to the body to use, and could explain why people who eat lots of nuts aren't necessarily overweight (although my guess is that people who eat lots of nuts are more likely to consumer a healthier diet overall diet). It's best to keep the nuts whole if you are trying to lose weight as ground nuts and nut butters are much more easily digested. Eating them with the skins on will provide an extra fibre boost.

How to buy and store

The fat in nuts becomes rancid over time and especially in warm conditions. To keep them fresh, buy nuts in smaller packs, enough for you to eat in three to four weeks. Seal the pack securely after you've used them and if you get a whiff of a paint-like smell or they taste bitter, chuck them out. Larger quantities are more economical, but consider keeping them in the fridge or freezer if there is space. To do this, divide them into smaller portions and store in airtight jars or lidded containers – you don't want any moisture to get in as it could attract mould or soften the nuts.

How to eat more

• Buy packs of mixed nuts and dried fruit (such as raisins and cranberries) for a healthy snack. The dried fruit will add the sweetness you may be missing from your usual treat.

- Make your own unsweetened muesli for breakfast (see recipe on page 234), or try a Swiss-style bircher muesli (page 237) for a change. Prepare just enough muesli to last for two weeks, so it doesn't get a chance to go stale. Top with thick bio yogurt with fresh berries, mixed nuts and a drizzle of runny honey for a probiotic and polyphenol-rich breakfast.
- Sprinkle nuts onto salads and blitz into dressings. Try serving chopped nuts scattered over lightly cooked green vegetables, and use nuts in your stir-fries too.
- Blitz nuts into chickpeas or beans for falafel and veggie burgers to help make the mixture thicker and easier to form. The addition of finely chopped onion and garlic will make your gut microbes even happier.
- Use nuts when you make cookies or flapjack-style bars. They will help to balance blood sugar levels and add extra nutrients.
- For an after-dinner treat, drizzle Brazil nuts with melted dark chocolate (no less than 70 per cent cocoa solids). Leave to set on a parchment-lined tray and serve with coffee.
- Serve warm roasted nuts as a snack, or make them into a satay-style sauce for dipping raw vegetables.

A word about calories

If we eat more calories than we burn, put on weight. It's a simple balancing act – or is it? New research is challenging the idea that the body will process a calorie from junk food, for example, in the same way that it would a calorie from an apple. Scientists have also pointed out that there are a number of factors which affect our real calorie intake, and what our bodies do with that energy. Food labelling isn't always accurate, and those with longer guts can extract more calories from the food they eat. The make-up of our gut flora is another factor at play in our blood sugar responses to food. Keeping an eye on calories is a useful guide to the energy density of food, but we should look at the source of that energy too, and ask what else it can give us.

CHOCOLATE

Cocoa contains over 300 chemicals, and researchers have sifted through many of them to identify the strong benefits of compounds called flavonoids. They're part of the same polyphenol family found in nuts and olives, which boasts anti-inflammatory, antioxidant and microbial effects.

Gram for gram, cocoa has the highest concentration of polyphenols and flavonoids of any food. In the gut, microbes seem to enjoy chocolate as much as we do, metabolising chemicals from cocoa in a variety of useful ways. Cocoa flavonoids used in research were seen to increase levels of good bifido and lactobacilli bacteria and reduce numbers of those from the firmicute family, which have been implicated in the rise of obesity. The fact that cocoa beans are fermented before roasting may be significant here.

Chocolate containing 70 per cent or more cocoa solids is rich, dark, slightly bitter and much better for us than a milkier, milder chocolate which may only contain around 26 per cent cocoa. Although milk chocolate uses the same type of cocoa as dark chocolate, to get the polyphenol benefits you would need to eat three to five times as much – bad news for your waistline. White chocolate doesn't contain any cocoa solids, so it offers more in the way of sugar and fat than polyphenols.

Think about incorporating a square of dark chocolate into your daily diet, and don't forget about cocoa powder – the unsweetened type is made from 100 per cent cocoa solids. Sticking to 25g or less a day should help you reap the benefits without piling on the pounds.

How to buy and store

Buy only chocolate containing at least 70 per cent cocoa solids. Eighty per cent is even better, and it's now possible (but perhaps not hugely appetising) to buy 100 per cent cocoa chocolate. Bear in mind that the more cocoa solids the chocolate contains, the more bitter it will taste, so a little will go a long way. There's a growing trend for raw chocolate, with accompanying claims that it's higher in flavonoids. It's also very expensive, so for now I'm happy to stick to the conventional chocolate that has been the subject of most of the research. But I do look out for mini bars of artisan chocolate made with proper cacao, which is the purest form of chocolate you can eat. It's far less processed than most cocoa powder or chocolate bars. Once open, keep your bar of choice tightly wrapped in a lidded container.

Some cocoa powder is treated with alkaline chemicals, or 'Dutched', during manufacture, which reduces its acidity and rounds out the flavour. Studies have shown that there are much lower flavonoid levels in Dutched cocoa. If you're looking for a flavonoid boost from your cocoa, check the label and choose one which doesn't list an acidity regulator.

If you might be tempted to eat too much at once, break it into squares and keep it in a lidded container in the freezer.

How to eat more

- Try finely grating dark chocolate onto a small bowl of thick bio yogurt and top with sliced just-ripe banana for a quick dessert which your microbes will love.
- Make proper hot chocolate by melting grated dark chocolate in semi-skimmed milk and adding a little unrefined sugar (such as light brown muscovado) to taste. You can also use good-quality cacao or cocoa powder. Add a little vanilla extract or warm spices such as cinnamon and you won't need quite as much sugar to sweeten it.
- Stir grated dark chocolate into freshly made porridge for a fibre and polyphenol-rich breakfast.
- Dip fresh strawberries into melted dark chocolate and leave to set. Serve as an informal dessert or fruity snack. Dip bananas into melted dark chocolate, sprinkle with chopped nuts and freeze on parchment-lined trays for a healthy summer choc ice.
- Stir chopped dark chocolate or non-Dutched cocoa powder into chilli con carne or braised beef or game casseroles. It will add richness and flavour as well as nutritional benefits.
- Let one square of chocolate melt very slowly on your tongue for as long as you can. Studies have shown that chocolate eaten this way before meals can help prevent you consuming too much. Eat it this way after a meal and you're also less likely to snack.

RED WINE

Recent findings from around 12,000 subjects participating in the American and British Gut Projects have shown an increase in microbial diversity in regular alcohol drinkers. Scientists believe that microbial diversity is very beneficial for our health.

Although the evidence is unclear, and many wine drinkers in the study also drank beer, there are other reasons to suspect that red wine may contain some chemical substances that could be healthy. Grapes are extremely rich in polyphenols, and at last count contained 109 healthy chemicals, including flavonoids and the super-trendy compound resveratrol.

Sometimes sold as a supplement, resveratrol is found in red grapes, peanuts and some berries. Studies have shown that it could offer a huge variety of advantages, such as increasing longevity and reducing heart disease, dementia and cancer. It has also been associated with helping reduce obesity, although less is known about how well it's absorbed, and you may have to consume unfeasible amounts to be useful.

There's more evidence for the benefits of red wine than for white, however, and spirits don't seem to have the same benefits, so should be avoided or drunk only occasionally. The latest research also shows that what we drink and what effect it has on us is very personal, due to our genes and also to our microbes.

How to buy and store

If you're going to drink red wine, avoid the cheapest bottles and choose those from smaller winemakers – you could even try 'natural' wines, which are made on a small scale with minimal intervention. Better wines are less processed and likely to contain more beneficial compounds; it's quality over quantity. Moderate wine consumption (perhaps one small glass a few days a week) is considered a good thing, and too much wine negates the benefits.

I also use red wine quite liberally in my cooking. Some research has shown that resveratrol isn't affected by heat, so I'm going to continue to use wine in dishes where it makes them all the more delicious and trust that it's keeping my microbes happy too.

Incredible as it might seem, as well as a dozen polyphenols, coffee also contains a surprisingly high amount of soluble fibre similar to the kind found in apples and oats. There's around half a gram in every cup, depending on the type of coffee. Soluble fibre aids digestion, helps the body absorb vital nutrients and helps keep cholesterol levels under control.

The combination of fibre and polyphenols means that coffee provides food for our gut microbes, so for most people a cup or two a day can be a beneficial part of eating for gut health. And while tea can't match coffee for fibre, green and black tea both contain flavonoids.

If you have a problem with caffeine, don't worry; the soluble fibre found in coffee is just as abundant in decaf. A medium-sized cup of takeaway coffee could hold the same amount of soluble fibre as an apple! And even freeze-dried instant coffee seems to contain it, alongside a decent dose of polyphenols. Because the good stuff in coffee seems to survive most processing, you can be guided by personal taste, but don't sweeten with sugar or syrups and remember, cream will add lots of calories with few other benefits.

How to buy and store

If you love coffee, it will be easy to drink a couple of cups a day. Many people find that having a cup first thing in the morning helps that early trip to the loo. Think about investing in a proper coffee maker – capsule machines are quick and mess-free and, at around 30p a cup, the coffee works out far cheaper than buying your brew from a coffee shop. It also means you can experiment with different varieties and strengths of coffee.

If you buy coffee destined for filters or cafetières, keep it in an airtight container once opened as the flavour will be lost when it is exposed to air.

How to drink more

- If you make your own cappuccino using coffee capsules and a milk frother, don't forget to sprinkle with cocoa powder to get extra antioxidant benefits. You can also stir cocoa powder into hot coffee for a mocha-style drink.

- Make choco-mocha pots for an occasional dessert by mixing melted dark chocolate with strong coffee and a touch of sugar, then blending with eggs and a little cream.
- Make a refreshing summer drink by whizzing cold strong coffee with full-fat bio yogurt, milk and ice cubes in a blender. Serve in tall glasses.

Did you know...

Total polyphenol content is more important than isolating different compounds and it is possible to increase your total intake substantially by eating more fruit. All fruits have useful polyphenol levels, but blueberries, strawberries, raspberries, grapes and apples are particularly good sources. Eat two to three servings a day for the maximum benefits. Whole fruit also contains lots of soluble fibre to help keep gut microbes well fed.

How to include greater diversity

It's easier to increase the diversity of your diet than you might think. Many foods are readily available in supermarkets and can be incorporated into your daily diet with very little faff.

PULSES

Pick up a mixed bag of dried pulses – containing a range of different legumes from beans to lentils – and you'll bring different flavours, colours and textures to your salads, stews and soups. Some mixed bags also contain wholegrains, such as barley, so you are getting even more diversity.

CANNED BEANS

Look for cans, jars or cartons of mixed beans to get the diversity you are looking for, or make your own mix then freeze what you aren't going to use immediately to add to a soup or stew. Avoid those canned with sugar, salt or sauces. Canned beans are cooked in the can, so the liquid may contain nutrients. You only need to rinse beans when using in a salad or to make burgers or falafel.

RICE

Brown rice and wholegrain rice are the same thing but packets can be labelled differently. It's possible to buy bags of mixed brown rice with red rice and wild rice which helps keep things interesting for your gut microbes. Wholegrain rice takes longer to cook, so bear in mind when you are planning a meal. I've found that the par-boiled and dried easy-cook wholegrain rices from brands such as Uncle Ben's are a brilliant storecupboard standby as the rice only takes 10 minutes. It sometimes comes packaged in boil-in-the-bags, which is useful for portion control. I also add diversity to my wholegrain rice by cooking broccoli or another vegetable in the same water as the rice – adding for the last few minutes – and then draining and tossing with a few nuts or seeds.

NUTS

It's easy to buy nuts in mixed bags, and some even have a few dried fruits or seeds tossed in. They're great for sprinkling onto salads, porridge or yogurt for breakfasts, soups or as a snack. Don't forget, though, that nuts are high in calories and eating huge quantities isn't a great idea. Just a small handful a day will help provide the nutrients and diversity that your gut microbes love.

SEEDS

Like nuts, it's easy to buy mixed bags of seeds. They usually contain a combination of pumpkin seeds, sunflower seeds and sesame seeds. Sometimes you'll find a pack containing linseeds too – an added bonus for diversity-seeking microbes. You can also mix your own seed combinations and keep in an airtight jar.

MUESLI

If you're a cereal fan, make up your own muesli. Make sure it has a really good variety of different cereals, nuts, seeds and dried fruit to benefit your gut. Keep it in an airtight jar.

FROZEN VEGETABLES

It's good to know that frozen vegetables are just as nutritious as fresh because they are harvested and frozen very quickly. If you freeze your own garden produce, make sure you do so on the day it is picked, in order to preserve as many nutrients as possible.

Bags of mixed frozen vegetables will give you diversity at an affordable price, so think about supplementing your fresh produce with frozen, especially during the winter months.

FROZEN FRUIT

Buying some fruit ready-frozen is a good idea as it tends to be more economical than stuffing the fridge with fresh fruit alone. A bowlful of frozen berries can be thawed in the fridge overnight, ready for topping yogurt or porridge in the morning. They can also be used for oaty crumbles, fruit tarts and, of course, smoothies.

MIXED LEAVES

Mixed leaves are another great way of getting a variety of different greens. They are more expensive than buying plain lettuce but the combination of leaves brings additional nutrients to your diet. If you have space, try growing your own. A windowsill is enough to keep a supply of baby leaves going through the summer. If you are buying from the supermarket, look out for leaves that are unwashed as they haven't been dunked in a sterilising bath before packing. Rinse them at home instead (ideally in filtered water).

BREAD AND CRACKERS

Choose wholegrain or seeded bread and you'll include an additional range of vitamin-rich grains and seeds in your daily mix, plus the extra fibre that your microbes will love. Wholegrain dark rye breads make a nice change and look out for naturally fermented sourdough bread too. All bread freezes well and slices don't take long to defrost, or can be toasted from frozen. I sometimes buy seeded crackers or sourdough crackers too. Look for those with a good mix of seeds and grains but stay away from any with lots of artificial additives. It's usually a case of spending a little more to get a better product, but they'll keep well in an airtight tin and can be enjoyed with any of your gut-happy platters.

A few foods to avoid

Emulsifiers

Try and stay away from any foods that contain emulsifiers, such as canned coconut milk (unless it is 100 per cent pure coconut milk) and shop-bought dressings. It has been shown that some emulsifiers, the ones used in ice cream manufacture particularly, bind with bacteria in your gut and effectively disable gut microbes from doing their job.

Sugars

Eliminating all sugar from our diets isn't achievable or desirable – you could tie yourself in knots trying to avoid it. But it is widely accepted that sugar, especially the sugar added to processed food and drink, has a lot to answer for in terms of the obesity epidemic and associated health problems. That's why you won't find a large amount of sweet things in this book, and most of them include fruit, whose sugar comes with a whole package of nutritional and prebiotic benefits.

We don't know an awful lot about how sugar affects gut bacteria, just that they're not well adapted to cope with large amounts of it. Refined sugar is apparently the biggest villain of the piece, but the 'natural' alternatives we're faced with – including coconut sugar and carob, agave, date and maple syrups – can be obscure and often expensive. I think it's useful to remember that the body processes all sugar in the same way, and that too much is bad for us. Choose an alternative sugar only if you prefer the taste of, say, honey or muscovado to the white stuff, but bear in mind that it still packs a calorific punch, and keep it to a minimum.

Artificial sweeteners are the subject of ongoing debate. They travel through the gut and arrive unaltered in the colon, where they can interact with gut microbes. Animal studies have found a reduction in gut microbes, especially healthy microbes, following a regime of sucralose consumption, and human studies have had similarly concerning results. If you can, it's a good idea to try to conquer a sweet tooth rather than replace sugar with sweeteners.

3| Living a gut-healthy lifestyle

Stay hydrated

Water is a crucial element of digestion, and fluid and fibre consumption should go hand in hand. If you boost your fibre intake (which should be done gradually) without drinking enough water, you are very likely to experience discomfort. If you are increasing your fibre intake, you will need to drink more, otherwise you will get constipated.

Water and us

Humans are 50–65% water; all our cells are bathed in and contain water. It is essential for many of the processes that keep us alive. Water is crucial for good physical and brain health. It helps our heart pump blood with less effort, maintains healthy skin elasticity and reduces the burden placed on our liver and kidneys, which need to rid our body of waste products. It maintains our ability to concentrate and think. We can live without food for a relatively long time, but water is essential.

The trouble is, we are constantly losing water, be it in our urine, poo, tears, sweat or breath. Digestion is a big water-grabber, which makes sense: we need water to keep the system moving and help remove our waste. But if we're running short on water in the rest of our bodies, the digestive system extracts more from our food, making poo harder and more difficult to pass. When we do lose water, we need to replenish it in order to stop us dehydrating.

Staying hydrated

You should drink when you feel thirsty, but current recommendations sit at the equivalent of around six to eight 200ml glasses of water a day (and that can include total liquids such as tea and coffee too). Your intake needs to match your loss of water so more is necessary if, for example, you are sweating after exercise. If you are increasing your fibre intake, you will need to drink more, otherwise you will get constipated.

Water is the best option for staying hydrated. As we're constantly being reminded, other drinks may add extra, empty calories to the diet. This is true of fruit juices as well as the classic fizzy drinks. However, any drink, including tea and coffee, is primarily water and therefore contributes to your levels of hydration. Don't forget that all food will contain some water, and a significant amount is contained in fruits and vegetables. Drinking water might also help to reduce feelings of hunger.

Getting enough water

- **Keep a bottle, jug or glass of water within reach. There is no need to spend money on bottled water, just fill up from the tap or water filter jug and decant as you need to. If you don't like plain water, you can add a little flavour with slices of lime, lemon or cucumber, perhaps with fresh mint.**
- **Have a drink of water with every meal, even if you've got a glass or mug of something else on the go. Drinking alongside a meal does not interfere with digestion.**
- **If you are exercising hard, make sure you drink before, during and after activity.**

Keep moving

Why you should add exercise to your daily routine

These days we have access to plenty of food and take in far more calories than we burn in a day sitting at a desk. This means we will store the extra calories consumed. The body has learnt to store things for a rainy day, the problem being that this might have worked well back in the Stone Age when food was not always plentiful, and still does work well in homes around the world where food is not always on hand, but it doesn't work well if there is never any 'rain' and the cupboards are always full. We just store more and more fat and risk becoming overweight or obese.

Fat changes the metabolism and cell signals in the body. This causes insensitivity of the body to the insulin hormone and the body then provides too much. Victims will suffer from type two diabetes, a disease with daily management issues, along with the potential for a multitude of complications.

Exercise and the gut

There's lots yet to explore about the links between exercise and the gut, but studies show a positive correlation between regular exercise and a healthy microbiome. In animal studies, scientists have identified a link between running and altered microbe composition, helping to strengthen immunity and dampen inflammation.

Exercise can also help with the wider function of the gut. We are constantly reminded that heart health suffers if we don't exercise it. Like any muscles in the body, the 'use it or lose it' rule applies. Muscle strength and endurance is built up over time, but is easily lost, and fitness extends to your gut too. Being upright is half the battle, as moving keeps your gut moving. Keep active to keep your gut active. Working the abdominal muscles in a rhythmic fashion (as when we walk about) can stimulate a bowel movement by increasing the blood flow to the gut, and triggering peristalsis. This contributes to the perfect poo (see page 67).

Without exercise our circulation is sluggish and tissues that are squashed or stretched by static posture struggle to get a good supply of blood. They then find it difficult to get rid of the waste products their cells want to expel. Exercise increases blood flow and moves the stretched tissues to slacken them off or release a tissue that is squashed, enabling the flushing out of these products around the body. That's good for just about everything.

Movement boosts happy hormones and chemicals, so we feel better after exercise. Add to that the sense of achievement if you have reached a goal, and exercise is an all-round tonic.

Exercise and the gut

- If you decrease exercise, your gut can slow down, too, leading to constipation. But if you're already taking enough exercise, adding more to your routine won't necessarily get things moving.
- Stress dampens digestion, slowing the process down and inhibiting the extraction of energy from food. Exercise helps beat everyday stress, adding another motivation to get moving.
- When you move more, you need to drink more. Increase your hydration levels in line with your exercise so that water isn't stolen from that perfect poo.

The perfect poo

It may not be a subject many of us relish, but the perfect poo can offer reassurance about your gut health and even elements of your general health.

The perfect poo has the right colour, the right consistency and the right diameter. It will arrive on time and with minimal effort. Once disposed of, life can go on comfortably without further thought.

A perfect poo is three-quarters water, which is needed to keep the poo soft enough to pass through your colon smoothly and efficiently, and explains why digestion is such a water-grabbing business. About a third of the remaining solids is made up of a mixture of dead and live bacteria from your gut, and another third is undigested plant-based fibre from things like fruit, vegetables, grains and pulses. The last bit contains mucus, digestive juices and broken-down blood cells, plus the remains of medicines and food colourings which need to be ejected from the body. It is these components that account for colour and consistency. Assuming the passage of poo is not interrupted by a narrowed or stretched inner tubing, the size should be about right for an optimal exit.

Colour

A shade of brown is normal, with or without a hint of yellow. Different colours, or those that are unusual for you, may indicate something is wrong. For example, if your gut bleeds inside, the blood will clot on its way out and create a black colour which needs to be investigated by your GP. Bleeding from piles (haemorrhoids) doesn't have time to clot and looks fresh; this is less worrying, but you should seek help if it's a new symptom. Other colours that should alert you to a possible problem are light brown to greyish-white (which may indicate a kink in your liver-gut connection) and pale yellowy-brown, which can be a sign of problems with your enzymes or gut bacteria, or part and parcel of an attack of diarrhoea or a course of antibiotics.

Consistency

The consistency and content of your poo also affect the density of it. The perfect poo will sink slowly and gently hit the bottom of the pan – it contains gas bubbles created by gut bacteria that give it a little buoyancy. If food is poorly digested and stools are hard and dehydrated, they will drop like a stone. If poo has a high content of undigested fat, it will float just like oil on water.

Diameter

Most of us have a fairly standard width to our poos. If you notice a change, particularly if your poos become more pencil-like, it might indicate a restriction somewhere. Seek help from your doctor.

Time

Most of us are fairly habitual about when we visit the loo, and after breakfast or the first meal of the day is common. Most of us go the same number of times a day each day: some people once, some twice, some only go every two days; if you tend to be constipated, you may go several days between each poo.

When you start the 28-day plan, your body may take a few days to get used to the increase in fibre. Once reawakened, you should find that you need to do a poo at least once a day. You will also find that your poos increase in size as the amount of undigested fibre in your gut grows. This shouldn't be a problem as your stools should remain soft enough to pass easily.

Watch out for changes in your habits that you struggle to explain. We all know that a change in diet, which might happen when we travel, can interfere with routines but once home things return to normal. If this fails to be the case, it's always worth discussing with your GP. You may feel embarrassed, but GPs talk about poo frequently and won't bat an eyelid – for them, it's just another diagnostic tool.

Does the way you sit on the loo make a difference?

The research would seem to say yes. Western loos, where the user sits, don't seem to be the best idea. Instead the French, along with many Asian countries, have adopted more effective habits. Here, squatting or similar positions facilitate passing a poo with greater ease. If you have ever had the misfortune of struggling with constipation, or were worried about the first poo after having had an abdominal operation or a baby, you might remember that having your knees up helped. Try resting your feet on a low stool or stack of books when you next have a poo and see if it moves things along – or try rocking forwards on the loo, which can really help.

Three tips to help keep things moving

- Raise your knees, as if you're squatting, when you do a poo. Use a small stack of books, low stool or upturned box to elevate your feet.
- If you're struggling with a poo, rocking forwards and back into an upright position a few times should help encourage things along.
- Keep your muscles healthy by exercising, so you stay in control.

Don't worry if you don't poo every day, especially towards the beginning of the plan. If your diet has been completely revamped, your gut will still be adjusting. As you eat more plant-based fibre, the volume and frequency of your poos will increase, as long as you remember to drink more fluids. Towards the end of the 28 days you should find that you are producing 'perfect' poos more frequently – definitely something to be proud of!

Avoid stress and eat mindfully

Stress

The gut is sensitive, and the most obvious link between stress and our stomachs is when, under extreme strain, stress or anxiety, we can't keep anything down. But studies show that more everyday stresses can also tax the gut. When the brain has a stress-related problem it needs to solve, it borrows energy from the gut and the blood supply usually available for digestion is reduced. The longer the stress continues, the more likely the gut is to react by causing loss of appetite or diarrhoea. There's also a theory that stress alters the balance of bacteria in the gut, allowing only the hardiest ones (which are not necessarily the friendliest) to survive.

Stress and anxiety can be difficult to predict and control, but if you follow my advice in the chapter on exercise, you'll be making a good start – exercise is great for keeping everyday problems in perspective and thinking through knotty issues. I also heard a bit of great advice which is given in some enlightened workplaces: if you have time, spend ten minutes outside. If you don't, spend twenty.

Sleep and routine

We all feel better when we're well rested, and so does our gut. As I said in Part One, giving your gut a break for a period of around twelve hours will help your stomach and small intestine finish their work effectively. You'll usually be asleep for lots of this important breaktime. This is another reason to prioritise sleep, so take the time to create a calm, quiet sleep environment and a pre-bed routine that works for you – and ban screens from the bedroom, if you can.

Sleep is an important part of our routine, and most guts thrive on knowing exactly what's coming. Travel disrupts this, with meals and sleep arriving at odd times and in different forms than usual – and the results can upset our digestion. If your routine changes, staying hydrated, getting whatever exercise you can and seeking out fresh, unprocessed foods with a decent fibre content can help. And if you need to go to the toilet, go.

Eating mindfully

This popular but vague term is a bit of a buzzword, but think about its opposite – eating mindlessly – and mindfulness starts to feel more helpful at the table. There's plenty of research to show that we eat more when we're distracted (a good reason to avoid eating in front of the TV or computer), and rushing through a meal is no way to treat a gut that appreciates a well-chewed mouthful. So take your time, and don't try to do anything else while you're eating.

Mindfulness is also useful when it comes to preparing and serving the dishes on this plan. Put together your meals with a bit of care, thinking about using a variety of ingredients and considering portion size, colour and contrast – it'll help you enjoy everything more without going off-plan.

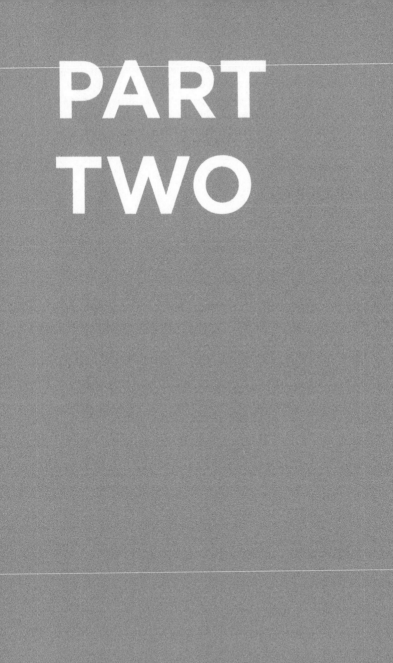

PART TWO

The 28-day healthy gut plan

How to use this plan

The aim of this eating plan is to help your body function more effectively. Research shows that by looking after your gut, you can reboot your health, lose weight and live longer. This plan provides plenty of ideas for meals brimming with the probiotics, prebiotics and polyphenols that will make your gut happy, but as we've seen, lifestyle is important too. I'd say that there are five steps to achieving gut nirvana.

- Eat a varied diet of fresh, unprocessed food, including lots of fruit and vegetables.
- Include plenty of probiotic fermented foods and fibre-rich prebiotic foods.
- Eat natural foods rich in polyphenol antioxidants, such as extra virgin olive oil.
- Avoid antibiotics unless absolutely necessary.
- Avoid stress, take exercise and eat mindfully.

The diversity diet

This plan follows proven ways to improve your health, such as the Mediterranean diet, and incorporates new ideas that have recently been shown to encourage microbe diversity and lead to weight loss, plus better health, energy and mood.

The Mediterranean diet is rich in plant-based foods such as vegetables, fruit, legumes (fresh beans and peas, dried beans and lentils) and wholegrains. It contains moderate amounts of chicken and fish, and a little red meat. Most of the fat is unsaturated and comes from foods such as extra virgin olive oil and nuts as well as saturated fats from cheese and yogurt. Having a small amount of red wine regularly is also thought to be beneficial to health.

Research has shown that this way of eating can improve weight loss, give better control of blood sugar levels and reduce the risk of depression. It has also been associated with reductions in levels of inflammation – a risk factor for heart attack, stroke and Alzheimer's disease.

The plan follows the Mediterranean way of eating, but there's no need to eat just Mediterranean-style dishes. I've created a huge variety of fibre-recipes which are based on the principles that make this a great way to eat, but have global influences. You'll find spicy Indian curries, Chinese stir-fries, vitamin and fibre-packed salads and Swiss mueslis, as well as some very British dishes, such as beef stew. The meal plan will make your diet more diverse than it has probably ever been, but it's so easy to follow that you're unlikely to notice just how many more foods you are eating.

How to make the plan work for you

Eating well for your gut is easy on my 28-day plan – just follow my suggestions for breakfast, lunch and dinner! But this isn't a conventional diet plan, and I've designed all the recipes so that, if you wish, you can mix things up between days and still stay firmly on the gut health wagon. I've designed the plan to help you lose weight – you could lose up to a stone in the four weeks. It's still a great way of eating even if you aren't looking to drop a few pounds, but you may need to increase the portion sizes a little or add a couple of healthy snacks.

Breakfast is a moveable feast which doesn't have to be eaten first thing. It is a chance to get some gut-healthy goodies inside you, though, and because you won't be overeating in the evening, you may rediscover an appetite for breakfast.

For lunch a few days of the week, you can expect to put together a gut-happy platter which will help you to get the diversity you need and include a variety of different vegetables, fruits, pulses and grains. Inspired by the enticingly colourful but highly priced deli lunches that are now available in many cafes and salad bars, these can be different every day and as exotic or familiar as you like. On other days, you can choose a salad or soup which is packed with similar benefits.

There is no need to eat at exactly the same time each day, or even have three meals a day. If at all possible, wait for your body to tell you that you are hungry, rather than filling up on snacks, however healthy they might be, or eating simply because that's your habit. A larger meal in the morning could mean it's several hours until your body is ready for lunch, or you might want to go right through to supper. By listening to your gut, you will definitely eat less overall, your body will be ready to accept the new food and your gut lining will be rested and ready to digest the next meal as efficiently as possible while allowing for a greater variety of microbes to flourish.

Pick and mix

With a variety of different ingredients to hand, you are going to create your own colourful, crunchy, vitamin and fibre-rich meals to help keep you full and your gut microbes happy.
You will find that once your body is treated to all the nutrients it could possibly wish for, your food cravings should start to disappear, your skin will glow and your energy will soar.

For the gut-happy platter, I have suggested a range of different prepared vegetables, dips, meats, fish, nuts, fruit and cheeses that you can have to hand in your fridge. All you need to do is gather a few of them – at least ten different ingredients – and put them on a plate or into a lidded lunch box if you are eating away from home. With the flexibility to choose your own lunch, you shouldn't have any waste at the end of the week. And because there are a range of bought and homemade foods that you can pick from, there is no need to ever go hungry or end up eating something that isn't going to benefit your gut.

My ten-plus salads contain a huge range of gut-healthy ingredients but are simple to prepare and can be eaten at home or taken to work. Some of these combinations can also be served warm, heated in a microwave or in a pan on the hob.

It's worth having at least two soups in the freezer, for colder days or when you really don't have any time for preparation. Sprinkle them with a variety of seeds or chopped nuts and serve a probiotic food alongside – this could be as simple as a large spoonful of live yogurt or something more exotic, such as kimchi or sauerkraut. You can serve these with wholegrain or sourdough bread if you like.

To make things extra simple, I've given lots of tips and ideas and you can see photos of some of the dishes in the middle section of this book and online at www.justinepattison.com.

Before you begin

Once you have committed to this way of eating, you should feel so much better, there will be no going back. Highly processed foods and meals without a huge amount of diversity may still be a temptation. The aim is to avoid these during your 28 days, but if you follow the rules most of the time, the occasional diversion won't undermine the plan.

The 28-day plan is quite a commitment, but once you get into the swing of things, you will find it very easy to follow.

The main meal suggestions I have given aren't set in stone, but I wanted to give you a selection of delicious dishes to choose from. If you work your way through the dishes as I have recommended, you will eat a huge variety of foods without having to spend hours planning. It also means that after the 28 days, you will have a tried and tested new repertoire of different meal ideas to enjoy.

I strongly recommend that you give your digestive system a break for around twelve hours each day. This will be mainly while you are asleep and means your gut can rest and rejuvenate with very little bother for you. It's a similar idea to intermittent fasting, which also works well for some people.

Clear the cupboards

In order to make room in your kitchen for all the gut-friendly foods you are going to be eating, it's a good idea to clear out your cupboards. I suggest you give away any crisps, biscuits, cakes and sweets that might tempt you. From now on, I'm going to refer to them as junk food. They are junk food because eating them in large quantities will make you feel rubbish. They don't have to be gone for good; if you really can't bear the thought of giving them away, put them in a lidded box, or even a small suitcase, and ask a friend to keep hold of them until the 28 days are up. I can guarantee that they won't hold any of their previous magical powers over you at the end of that time. In fact, after keeping off sugary foods and artificially seasoned snacks for 28 days, you will probably find them very unappetising.

Your body knows what it needs, it just requires a little time for your brain to kick into gear and help out. Everyone is different, but when the 28 days are up, your body, brain and gut microbes should be working far more harmoniously and the huge benefits that you will have felt should help keep you on track for life! Bear in mind that it can take several months of maintaining your weight loss until your body resets itself and automatically helps you stay at the new lower weight. Use the knowledge that you've learnt following the plan to inform your diet every day of your life, not just for the next few weeks.

Get well prepared

- Give your fridge and freezer a good clean-out, ready for the new foods that you will be keeping in there. Recycle or give away any old jars of sauces or half-opened packets of food. This is a fresh, new start and there needs to be space for all the delicious foods you are going to be eating.
- Write your shopping list for store cupboard ingredients that you don't already have, and the fresh foods you're going to buy. Don't put anything you don't need in your trolley.
- How far you plan ahead depends on your lifestyle, storage options and how often you shop, but it can be useful to aim to stock up on everything you need for the next three days.
- Decide which day you are going to start the plan and put aside some time the day before for preparation of things like sprinkles, dips and dressings and the makings of your chosen lunch platters. Having everything ready will really help you stick to the regime.
- Gather yourself a good selection of different-sized lidded plastic containers that can be used in the fridge or freezer. These don't have to be brand new; you may be able to reuse old takeaway containers or borrow some Tupperware from friends and family. Check out the selection in discount stores as they can be cheap and plentiful.
- Buy some good zip-seal freezer bags of different sizes for freezing any foods that you prepare in bulk.

- Get some sticky labels and a permanent marker for labelling the food in your fridge and freezer. And also for marking jars with the date of opening (something I always do which really helps me use up ingredients before their best-before date).

Make it easy for yourself

It's probably best to start the plan at the beginning of the week. If you start on a Monday, you will have the weekend for shopping and preparing ingredients for the following week. In just one hour, you could have enough lunches to take you through to Wednesday or even Thursday, if you make a couple of soups, too.

Bear in mind, too, that a big change in your eating patterns can mean your body needs a little time to adjust. If you aren't used to eating high-fibre foods, such as beans, other pulses plus lots of vegetables and fruit, you may need to take it easy for the first few days and then slowly increase the amounts. You will know if your body is finding the adjustment a bit sudden if you experience bloating or lots of wind. A bit of farting is fine and to be expected, but if things are getting uncomfortable, ease off a bit and then gradually increase your intake of the new foods.

Keep all the diversity in there if you can, but reduce the amounts. If a recipe calls for a whole can of beans and you have a few concerns, just use half or a third of the amount and freeze the rest. You'll find lots of freezing tips at the end of this book (page 298) so don't worry if you are unfamiliar with the process.

How to get the most out of the plan

When you are following the 28-day plan, I've made suggestions for gut-happy platters, soups and salads for the first week's menu. After that, you should be in the swing of things and able to choose your own lunchtime meals for the following three weeks. I've designed it like this to give you the flexibility to choose your lunch according to the weather, what you have in the fridge, how busy you are and what you feel like eating. You can also create your own salads using exactly the same principles as for the gut-happy platters (page 126). With just a little thought, you should be able to use up ingredients and leftovers for other meals very easily too, so there should be no wasted food on this plan. For instance, cooked chicken from a Sunday roast can be used for a salad or gut-happy platter on the Monday, half a can of beans, assorted leaves, or a few chunks of cheese can be incorporated into a salad and all sorts of vegetables can be combined and served alongside any of the main meal ideas.

To make sure you are getting enough diversity in your daily meals, jot down the ingredients you use for your lunches and any snacks. Make sure you are eating at least twenty different ingredients a day – it's actually surprisingly easy. Don't worry about listing every tiny bit of seasoning; stick with the main ingredients, such as different vegetables, beans, pulses, grains, meat and fish.

Because I recognise that many of us don't have much time to spend in the kitchen, I occasionally call for ready-made ingredients in place of home-cooked foods. I strongly feel that in order to eat well, a plan needs to fit with your lifestyle. If you are working long hours, have a young family or a busy lifestyle, or simply don't like or feel terribly confident about cooking, I need to make things as simple as possible for you. You'll find no fussy cooking methods here and the ingredient preparation is all pretty simple.

Sometimes I'll call for an ingredient, such as homemade flatbreads, but if you don't have time to make them, don't worry, buy the ready-made kind instead – I'll always give you an alternative. I also save time and money by using ready-made curry pastes on occasion. Just one jar of curry paste will last you a whole month, and saves spending on lots of individual spices. And you will be eating such a variety of wholesome, healthy foods that the occasional bought ingredient won't matter a bit. This healthy eating plan is meant to be a joy, not a trial.

This handbook has been designed to be wholly interactive, which means it's your book to write in – not just read from one end to the other and then forget about. It's a tool that you should have with you every day; one you can dip into any time to find a snippet of information or to log your progress. A combination of a diary and an information-rich guide.

On each page you'll find space to write and there are also tick boxes to encourage you to adjust your lifestyle and nourish your gut. It takes a while to break a habit, but keeping a daily record of actions and feelings is a great way to stay on course. Writing about your feelings might not come naturally, but it really does work – and you'll have the chance to see how far you have come.

SOMETHING NEW

This is simply a space to log anything that you might not have experienced before. It could be a new food you hadn't tried previously, or perhaps a recipe that you have prepared that you would never have considered making in the past. It's also a place that you can record feelings. You might want to say how great it is to be able to comfortably do up the zip on your trousers or that you had a great night's sleep for the first time in months. It might be having a spring in your step on the way to work, clearer skin or passing the newsagent's without craving crisps or chocolate. Anything that you think could make a difference to your success on the plan is worth writing down.

ACTIVITY

This is where you can record any sort of exercise you have completed. It might be a brisk walk to and from the shops, or a country amble. You may have done a session at the gym or taken part in a group sport. Vigorous housework, a spot of gardening or taking the stairs instead of the lift count, too. No matter what it is, just log the amount of time spent on the activity here. Aim for at least thirty minutes of activity five times a week, and more if possible.

Now, turn the page for your very own 28-day meal plan...

Wk 1	MEAL ONE	MEAL TWO	MEAL THREE
DAY 1	Yogurt and fruit with oat and nut crunch (page 234)	Gut-happy platter, Ten-plus salad or Soup	Veggie bolognese with spaghetti (page 212) Large mixed salad
DAY 2	Overnight muesli with berries (page 237)	Green pea and spinach soup (page 142)	Pan-fried pesto chicken (page 155) Large mixed salad
DAY 3	Boiled eggs with smoked salmon and asparagus soldiers (page 238)	Gut-happy platter, Ten-plus salad or Soup	Smoky bean chilli (page 216) Zingy avocado salsa (page 269) Fresh tomato salsa (page 268)
DAY 4	Yogurt and fruit with oat and nut crunch (page 234)	Gut-happy platter, Ten-plus salad or Soup	Simple soy and ginger salmon (page 195) Simple vegetable stir-fry (page 282)
DAY 5	Hot or cold oats (page 236)	Gut-happy platter, Ten-plus salad or Soup	Mixed vegetable and lentil curry (page 222) Fresh tomato salsa (page 268) Minted yogurt with cucumber (page 270)
DAY 6	Apple pancakes with blueberries and bananas (page 244)	Minestrone soup (page 140)	Steak and sweet potato wedges with blue cheese sauce (page 186) Simple gut-happy salad (page 271)
DAY 7	Mediterranean brunch eggs (page 241)	Chicken with 30 cloves of garlic (page 169) Spinach and potato mash (page 281) Five-plus mixed veg (page 277)	Weekend cheese platter (page 132)

Wk 2	MEAL ONE	MEAL TWO	MEAL THREE
DAY 8	Yogurt and fruit with oat and nut crunch (page 234)	Gut-happy platter, Ten-plus salad or Soup	Mediterranean vegetable lasagne (page 228) Large mixed salad
DAY 9	Overnight muesli with berries (page 237)	Gut-happy platter, Ten-plus salad or Soup	Pan-fried pork (or chicken) with apple and leek (page 184) Five-plus mixed veg (page 277)
DAY 10	Poached egg with smashed avocado (page 239)	Gut-happy platter, Ten-plus salad or Soup	Shepherdess pie (page 214) Five-plus mixed veg (page 277)
DAY 11	Yogurt and fruit with oat and nut crunch (page 234)	Gut-happy platter, Ten-plus salad or Soup	Italian fish stew (page 201) Warm beans with garlic and lemon (page 284) Yogurt mayonnaise (page 294)
DAY 12	Hot or cold oats (page 236)	Gut-happy platter, Ten-plus salad or Soup	Green vegetable and barley risotto (page 226) Large mixed salad
DAY 13	Scrambled eggs with asparagus (page 240)	Gut-happy platter, Ten-plus salad or Soup	Cheat's chicken tikka masala (page 161) Minted yogurt with cucumber (page 270) Fresh tomato salsa (page 268) Broccoli and almond rice (page 279)
DAY 14	Lower-sugar plum freezer jam (page 245) Yogurt cheese (page 246)	Quick roast lamb with mint (page 178)	Weekend cheese platter (page 132)

Wk 3	MEAL ONE	MEAL TWO	MEAL THREE
DAY 15	Yogurt and fruit with oat and nut crunch (page 234)	Gut-happy platter, Ten-plus salad or Soup	One-pan pasta with broccoli and tomatoes (page 210) Large mixed salad
DAY 16	Overnight muesli with berries (page 237)	Gut-happy platter, Ten-plus salad or Soup	One-pan chicken and tray bake (page 163)
DAY 17	Boiled eggs with smoked salmon and asparagus (page 238)	Gut-happy platter, Ten-plus salad or Soup	Sweet potato and spinach dhal (page 224) Minted yogurt with cucumber (page 270) Fresh tomato salsa (page 268)
DAY 18	Yogurt and fruit with oat and nut crunch (page 234)	Gut-happy platter, Ten-plus salad or Soup	Baked fish with fennel and smashed potatoes (page 198) Large mixed salad
DAY 19	Hot or cold oats (page 236)	Gut-happy platter, Ten-plus salad or Soup	Veg-packed peppers (page 215) Large mixed salad
DAY 20	Mediterranean brunch eggs (page 241)	Gut-happy platter, Ten-plus salad or Soup	Lamb and sweet potato tagine (page 180) Minted cucumber yogurt (page 270) Wholegrain rice, bulgur wheat or barley couscous
DAY 21	Apple pancakes with blueberries and bananas (page 244)	Roast Chicken with savoury rice (page 171) Large mixed salad or Five-plus mixed veg (page 277)	Weekend cheese platter (page 132)

Wk 4	MEAL ONE	MEAL TWO	MEAL THREE
DAY 22	Yogurt and fruit with oat and nut crunch (page 234)	Gut-happy platter, Ten-plus salad or Soup	Mediterranean vegetable lasagne (page 228) Large mixed salad
DAY 23	Overnight muesli with berries (page 237)	Gut-happy platter, Ten-plus salad or Soup	Lemony chicken stir-fry (page 157) Wholegrain rice or noodles
DAY 24	Poached eggs with smashed avocado (page 239)	Gut-happy platter, Ten-plus salad or Soup	Smoky bean chilli (page 216) Zingy avocado salsa (page 268) Fresh tomato salsa (page 269)
DAY 25	Yogurt and fruit with oat and nut crunch (page 234)	Gut-happy platter, Ten-plus salad or Soup	One-pan baked fish (page 193)
DAY 26	Hot or cold oats (page 236)	Gut-happy platter, Ten-plus salad or Soup	Mixed vegetable and lentil curry (page 222) Fresh tomato salsa (page 268) Minted yogurt with cucumber (page 270)
DAY 27	Leek and cheese omelette (page 243)	Gut-happy platter, Ten-plus salad or Soup	Sticky barbecue chicken (page 167) Large mixed salad or Rainbow coleslaw (page 272)
DAY 28	Lower-sugar plum freezer jam (page 245) Yogurt cheese (page 246)	Roast beef with shallots and red wine gravy (page 189) Five-plus mixed veg (page 277)	Weekend cheese platter (page 132)

Week 1 | **DAY 1**

Menu

Yogurt and fruit with oat and nut crunch (page 234) ☐

Gut-happy platter (page 126),
Ten-plus salad (page 248) or Soup ☐

Veggie bolognese with spaghetti (page 212) ☐

Large mixed salad ☐

Activity

. . . .

. . . .

. . . .

Something new

. . . .

. . . .

. . . .

Tip

Well done for making the commitment to starting the 28-day plan. At the end of it your body will be far in better balance, your energy levels will be soaring and you could have lost up to 14 pounds. Hopefully you will have plenty of food prepped for the week ahead and be ready to start! Don't forget to fill in any boxes on the pages that follow. Most of all, enjoy exploring all the different foods you will be preparing – your microbes will thank you for it.

Week 1 | DAY 2

Menu

Overnight muesli with berries (page 237) ☐

Gut-happy platter (page 126),
Ten-plus salad (page 248) or Soup ☐

Pan-fried pesto chicken (page 155) ☐

Large mixed salad ☐

Activity

....
....
....

Something new

....
....
....

Notes

....
....
....
....
....

Menu

Boiled eggs with smoked salmon and asparagus soldiers □
(page 238)

Gut-happy platter, Ten-plus salad or Soup □

Smoky bean chilli (page 216) □

Zingy avocado salsa (page 269) □

Fresh tomato salsa (page 268) □

Activity

....
....
....

Something new

....
....

Tip

Remember to keep your diet as diverse as possible. Research has
shown that many foods don't work as well nutritionally when they
are served in isolation. Spinach and carrots are good examples
because the nutrient carotene that they contain is better absorbed
into the body when they are served with the fat in an olive oil
dressing. Try to mix things up as much as possible.

Week 1 | DAY 4

Menu

Yogurt and fruit with oat and nut crunch (page 234) ☐

Gut-happy platter, Ten-plus salad or Soup ☐

Simple soy and ginger salmon (page 195) ☐

Simple vegetable stir-fry (page 282) ☐

Activity

....
....
....

Something new

....
....
....

Notes

....
....
....
....
....
....

Week 1 | DAY 5

Menu

Hot or cold oats (page 236) ☐

Gut-happy platter, Ten-plus salad or Soup ☐

Mixed vegetable and lentil curry (page 222) ☐

Fresh tomato salsa (page 268) ☐

Minted yogurt with cucumber (page 270) ☐

Activity

....

....

....

Something new

....

....

....

Tip

Don't forget to chew your food properly. It's easy when you're rushing or feeling really hungry to bypass the chewing and almost swallow things whole. Apart from increasing the risk of choking, swallowing food that is barely chewed and not adequately broken down makes it harder to absorb further down the track. So try to get into the habit now.

Week 1 | DAY 6

Menu

Apple pancakes with blueberries and bananas
(page 244) ☐

Minestrone soup (page 140) ☐

Steak with sweet potato wedges and blue cheese sauce
(page 186) ☐

Simple gut-happy salad (page 271) ☐

Activity

....
....
....

Something new

....
....
....

Notes

....
....
....
....

Menu

Mediterranean brunch eggs (page 241) ☐

Chicken with 30 cloves of garlic (page 169) ☐

Spinach and potato mash (page 281) ☐

Five-plus mixed veg (page 277) ☐

Weekend cheese platter (page 132) ☐

Activity

....

....

....

Something new

....

....

....

Tip

Think about what you have done over the last week and what you could improve next week – perhaps a way to make life a bit easier. Why not try ordering online, or buy differently? Perhaps you are preparing too much or could be freezing more?

Menu

Yogurt and fruit with oat and nut crunch (page 234) ☐

Gut-happy platter (page 126),
Ten-plus salad (page 248) or Soup ☐

Mediterranean vegetable lasagne (page 228) ☐

Large mixed salad ☐

Activity

....
....
....

Something new

....
....
....

Notes

....
....
....
....
....

Menu

Overnight muesli with berries (page 237) ☐

Gut-happy platter (page 126),
Ten-plus salad (page 248) or Soup ☐

Pan-fried pork (or chicken) with apple and leek
(page 184) ☐

Five-plus mixed veg (page 277) ☐

Activity

....

....

....

Something new

....

....

....

Tip

Keep on experimenting with your new food choices this week,
for instance by adding a couple of different ingredients to your
'Gut-happy platter'. Think about trying a different dip, perhaps
baba ganoush or olives stuffed with garlic cloves. Maybe some
nuts you haven't tried before.

Menu

Poached egg with smashed avocado (page 239) ☐

Gut-happy platter (page 126),
Ten-plus salad (page 248) or Soup ☐

Shepherdess pie (page 214) ☐

Five-plus mixed veg (page 277) ☐

Activity

....
....
....

Something new

....
....
....

Notes

....
....
....
....
....

Menu

Yogurt and fruit with oat and nut crunch (page 234) ☐

Gut-happy platter (page 126),
Ten-plus salad (page 248) or Soup ☐

Italian fish stew (page 201) ☐

Warm beans with garlic and lemon (page 284) ☐

Yogurt mayonnaise (page 294) ☐

Activity

....
....
....

Something new

....
....
....

Tip

Don't worry about eating the occasional food that's off-plan,
such as a takeaway meal, a cream cake or a bar of chocolate – as
long as you take your time eating it and really enjoy it, there is
no problem. As long as you are eating well most of the time, your
digestion will forgive you and your energy levels will remain high.

Week 2 | DAY 12

Menu

Hot or cold oats (page 236) ☐

Gut-happy platter (page 126),
Ten-plus salad (page 248) or Soup ☐

Green vegetable and barley risotto (page 226) ☐

Large mixed salad ☐

Activity

....
....
....

Something new

....
....
....

Notes

....
....
....
....
....

Menu

Scrambled eggs with asparagus (page 240) ☐

Gut-happy platter (page 126), ☐
Ten-plus salad (page 248) or Soup

Cheat's chicken tikka masala (page 161) ☐

Minted yogurt with cucumber (page 270) ☐

Fresh tomato salsa (page 268) ☐

Broccoli and almond rice (page 279) ☐

Activity

....
....
....

Something new

....
....

Tip

Make sure you are getting enough sleep. Research has shown that regular sleep deprivation puts the hormones that regulate appetite and metabolism out of sync, which may lead to weight gain and food cravings.

Week 2 | **DAY 14**

Menu

Lower-sugar plum freezer jam (page 245) ☐

Yogurt cheese (page 246) ☐

Quick roast lamb with mint (page 178) ☐

Weekend cheese platter (page 132) ☐

Activity

....
....
....

Something new

....
....
....

Notes

....
....
....
....
....
....

Menu

Yogurt and fruit with oat and nut crunch (page 234) ☐

Gut-happy platter (page 126),
Ten-plus salad (page 248) or Soup ☐

One-pan pasta with broccoli and tomatoes (page 210) ☐

Large mixed salad ☐

Activity

....

....

....

Something new

....

....

....

Tip

If you know you have a busy time coming up, why not make one
of your favourite recipes again and get the extra portions in the
freezer? Pack into individual servings so you can heat up quickly
and are never short of a gut-healthy meal. Stews, curries, chillies
and soups all freeze well.

Week 3 | **DAY 16**

Menu

Overnight muesli with berries (page 237) ☐

Gut-happy platter (page 126),
Ten-plus salad (page 248) or Soup ☐

One-pan chicken and tray bake (page 163) ☐

Activity

....
....
....

Something new

....
....
....

Notes

....
....
....
....
....
....

Menu

Boiled eggs with smoked salmon and asparagus soldiers ☐
(page 238)

Gut-happy platter (page 126), ☐
Ten-plus salad (page 248) or Soup

Sweet potato and spinach dhal (page 224) ☐

Minted yogurt with cucumber (page 270) ☐

Fresh tomato salsa (page 268) ☐

Activity

....
....
....

Something new

....
....
....

Tip

Today, think about embracing change. Think about the plan as
something to enjoy rather than a trial to endure. Imagine how
much better you are going to feel – you are probably noticing
changes in your health already. Reflect on them and perhaps write
down a difference that you have noticed in 'Something new'.

Week 3 | DAY 18

Menu

Yogurt and fruit with oat and nut crunch (page 234) ☐

Gut-happy platter (page 126),
Ten-plus salad (page 248) or Soup ☐

Baked fish with fennel and smashed potatoes (page 198) ☐

Large mixed salad ☐

Activity

....
....
....

Something new

....
....
....

Notes

....
....
....
....
....

Menu

Hot or cold oats (page 236) ☐

Gut-happy platter (page 126),
Ten-plus salad (page 248) or Soup ☐

Veg-packed peppers (page 215) ☐

Large mixed salad ☐

Activity

....
....
....

Something new

....
....
....

Tip

Keep an eye on portion sizes – especially of starchy carbs, such as
rice and pasta, even if they are wholegrain. It's easy for amounts to
climb up without you really noticing. If you want to lose weight, it's
best not to eat more than you could hold in one hand.

Week 3 | **DAY 20**

Menu

Mediterranean brunch eggs (page 241) ☐

Gut-happy platter (page 126),
Ten-plus salad (page 248) or Soup ☐

Lamb and sweet potato tagine (page 180) ☐

Minted cucumber yogurt (page 270) ☐

Wholegrain rice, bulgur wheat or barley couscous ☐

Activity

....
....
....

Something new

....
....
....

Notes

....
....
....
....

Menu

Apple pancakes with blueberries and banana (page 244) ☐

Roast chicken with savoury rice (page 171) ☐

Large mixed salad or Five-plus mixed veg (page 277) ☐

Weekend cheese platter (page 132) ☐

Activity

....

....

....

Something new

....

....

....

Tip

Take a photograph of your favourite meal of the day on your smartphone, or add some notes to the recipe about why you enjoyed it and what you might tweak – more herbs or a handful of olives? Plan to cook it again for friends and family and get their gut microbes going too.

Week 4 | **DAY 22**

Menu

Yogurt and fruit with oat and nut crunch (page 234) ☐

Gut-happy platter (page 126),
Ten-plus salad (page 248) or Soup ☐

Mediterranean vegetable lasagne (page 228) ☐

Large mixed salad ☐

Activity

....
....
....

Something new

....
....
....

Notes

....
....
....
....
....

Menu

Overnight muesli with berries (page 237) ☐

Gut-happy platter (page 126),
Ten-plus salad (page 248) or Soup ☐

Lemony chicken stir-fry (page 157) ☐

Wholegrain rice or noodles ☐

Activity

....
....
....

Something new

....
....
....

Tip

You are nearly at the end of the plan but it's important to stay
focused. Think about all the wonderful food you have been eating
and jot down a few of your favourite recipes in the notes section
of these pages as a reminder for the future.

Week 4 | **DAY 24**

Menu

Poached eggs with smashed avocado (page 239) ☐

Gut-happy platter (page 126),
Ten-plus salad (page 248) or Soup ☐

Smoky bean chilli (page 216) ☐

Fresh tomato salsa (page 268) ☐

Zingy avocado salsa (page 269) ☐

Activity

....
....
....

Something new

....
....
....

Notes

....
....
....
....

Menu

Yogurt and fruit with oat and nut crunch (page 234) ☐

Gut-happy platter (page 126),
Ten-plus salad (page 248) or Soup ☐

One-pan baked fish (page 193) ☐

Activity

....
....
....

Something new

....
....
....

Tip

You are now more than three weeks into the plan. Things should be working well and you should be getting used to this new way of eating. Why not give one of the more unusual probiotics a try? Think about adding kefir or kombucha to your daily menu. You can buy starter kits online and many health food stores sell the ready-made kind.

Week 4 | DAY 26

Menu

Hot or cold oats (page 236) ☐

Gut-happy platter (page 126),
Ten-plus salad (page 248) or Soup ☐

Mixed vegetable and lentil curry (page 222) ☐

Minted yogurt with cucumber (page 270) ☐

Fresh tomato salsa (page 268) ☐

Activity

....
....
....

Something new

....
....
....

Notes

....
....
....
....

Menu

Leek and cheese omelette (page 243) ☐

Gut-happy platter (page 126),
Ten-plus salad (page 248) or Soup ☐

Sticky barbecue chicken (page 167) ☐

Large mixed salad or Rainbow coleslaw (page 272) ☐

Activity

....
....
....

Something new

....
....
....

Tip

Well done for reaching the end of the plan! By now you should
be feeling full of energy and several pounds lighter. Get in touch
via www.justinepattison.com and let me know how you've got
on. Continue cooking and preparing your food the gut-happy
way once the 28 days are up. Or you could start right back at the
beginning and work your way through the menus again!

Menu

Lower-sugar plum freezer jam (page 245) ☐

Yogurt cheese (page 246) ☐

Roast beef with shallots and red wine gravy (page 189) ☐

Five-plus mixed veg (page 277) ☐

Weekend cheese platter (page 132) ☐

Activity

....
....
....

Something new

....
....
....

Notes

....
....
....
....
....

What's next?

I hope you've enjoyed using the *The Healthy Gut Handbook* as much as I've enjoyed writing it. As my family and I have progressed through the plan, trying out each recipe (and many more that we didn't have room for here), our way of eating has changed. It's given us more energy, better skin and a healthier outlook. We've lost weight where we needed to, are eating a wider diversity of foods than we ever did before and feel more in tune with our insides. I'm willing to bet that our gut microbes are pretty happy, too.

So, what's next? Research into the fascinating world of the human microbiome is continuing, and I'll be keeping an eye on how new studies continue to inform the ways we eat for gut health.

Personalised nutrition is an interesting area. Each and every human microbiome is different, meaning that we react to probiotics and prebiotics in very different ways. Looking at personal gut microbes is one way of working out what might help us lose weight or reduce inflammation, and the idea of tailoring your diet to suit your gut flora is a fascinating one which could alter our approach to diet and nutrition forever.

Get involved

If you are interested in looking more closely at your own microbiome, consider joining two projects run by Tim Spector from King's College London. The first is the British Gut Project – a huge open-source study of the human microbiome and its infinite variety. Participants make a small contribution to the project and send in a sample (which simply involves swabbing some used toilet paper), which is analysed for gut bacteria. You get to view the summary results online after 3–6 months but without any interpretation. If you want a more personalised commercial service join the MapMyGut service that Tim helped set up. Both projects are advancing this exciting branch of science linking our diet to differences in our gut microbes, health and our individuality.

You can find the microbe projects that best suit you by visiting the websites below.

www.britishgut.org
www.mapmygut.com

I also recommend reading Tim Spector's book, *The Diet Myth* for more details. Follow him on Twitter @timspector to keep up to date in this fast-moving area.

I hope you've discovered some favourite recipes that you'll cook again and again. You'll now know enough about gut-happy eating to adapt your own favourite recipes to boost their gut-happy credentials. But I also hope that you've developed new, healthy habits and an appetite for a diverse range of foods that's become second nature. You'll know that eating a colourful variety of plant-based foods is a great rule of thumb. You can, of course, turn back to this handbook any time you need ideas and inspiration.

And, if you want to see how many of these dishes looked while I was cooking them up in my test kitchen, have a browse on my website www.justinepattison.com for plenty of gut-happy recipe photos. You can also follow me on Instagram @justinepattison – I would love to hear how you get on, so do get in touch.

Frequently asked questions

I'm on the move all day, what should I do about lunch?

Pack a home-made salad containing a variety of different ingredients – around 10 is good. It doesn't need to be complicated, a selection of raw and cooked vegetables, legumes (such as beans and lentils), wholegrains, fruit, nuts and seeds, with an olive oil or yogurt dressing should be enough to keep you going. A hot soup or stew in a flask, with a serving of wholegrain bread, is good on a cold day. Don't forget that most supermarkets, and even petrol stations these days, also sell a selection of salads and dips that can be bought for immediate consumption. Pick those with the largest variety of wholesome ingredients, and avoid any with thick mayonnaise-style dressings and additives, such as emulsifiers and preservatives. If you aren't feeling hugely hungry, a pot of natural yogurt, some fresh fruit and mixed nuts will probably be enough.

I still feel hungry between meals, what should I do?

When your body is adjusting to eating differently, or less, you may feel hungry occasionally. It's a good idea to tune into this hunger and eat accordingly. I've recommended no more than three meals a day – but two might work better for you if you are aiming to lose weight. If you do feel hungry between meals, you can eat some fruit, vegetable sticks and perhaps a high-fibre bean-based dip, or a small handful of nuts. Phasing out regular snacking will help with the weight loss process and give your body time to absorb nutrients from your last meal and prepare for the next. Some people, especially those with manual jobs or an intensive exercise routine, may need to eat larger quantities more regularly. If this is the case, opt for more cooked root vegetables, extra wholegrains and pulses with your meals, increase protein and snack on fruit and nuts, and avoid fatty – or sugary – highly processed meals or snacks.

I've noticed that most of your recipes make two servings, but I want to cook for our whole family, what should I do?

Don't worry, all the recipes are easy to double or triple. I've designed the plan for two people to help make it easier to follow, but there is no reason why it can't be adapted for the whole family, especially the evening meals. You may need to use larger pans and increase some of the cooking times slightly, but the rest should be simple to calculate. You can always mix and match the ingredients and recipes according to what you think your family will eat, simply bearing in mind that the more variety and fibre, the better.

I love vegetarian foods but my partner needs more convincing. How can I encourage them to eat more veg and pulses?

I suggest that for the first week or two, you simply add more fibre in the form of lentils, beans or vegetables to your usual repertoire of recipes. If following the 28-day plan, add extra meat or poultry to the vegetarian dishes, such as a small portion of minced beef to the veggie bolognese, and include cooked meat or poultry in the salads at lunchtime. Also, reduce your meat serving size; buy smaller steaks or joint for roasting than you normally would, or cook one lamb chop instead of two. Bulk up the rest of the meal with plant-based foods and include plenty of protein-rich legumes.

I never eat breakfast, does that matter?

Don't worry about it. There's no need to eat breakfast unless you want to. You may find you are hungry later on in the morning, so have something to eat then or opt for an earlier lunch. Live yogurt, fruit, nuts and seeds are good foods to have on standby in case you start to feel peckish. If you are in a rush, or staying away from home, it's possible to pick a breakfast cereal that contains wholegrains and no added sugar. You'll need to look carefully at the label to check for added ingredients but these days there is quite a lot of choice, from no-added sugar mueslis to wholegrain shredded wheat, and a host of other cereals with tiny amounts of added sugar or salt. It might be worth whizzing up a simple home-made smoothie with live yogurt, milk, banana, berries and a few oats and nuts. Shop-bought smoothies can be laden with sugars, so it's best to make your own.

I'm going to a restaurant with friends tonight, what can I eat?

Eating out needn't be difficult. Look out for so-called superfood salads, which are likely to contain a good variety of fibre rich ingredients, or choose plainly cooked poultry, meat or fish with a large mixed salad or vegetable selection. If there really isn't anything you fancy, pick a meal you are going to enjoy, eat it without worrying and top up with healthier foods the next day. The occasional splurge isn't going to wreck your microbiome and could even add a bit of diversity to your diet depending on what you eat.

Should I always buy organic ingredients?

I'd say that it's important for your gut microbes to avoid food that's been subjected to lots of pesticides or antibiotics and look for ingredients with as few added chemicals as possible. This food is likely to be organic, or wild, so choose this when you can, and according to your budget, for the most health benefits.

Should I peel my vegetables before cooking or eating raw?

Peeling vegetables, such as potatoes and carrots, gets rid of a layer of fibre and vitamins that could benefit your gut microbes as well as your general health. If you are using organic vegetables and fruit, it's best to keep the skin on. I tend to scrub my vegetables really well and rinse in plenty of clean water before using, but you may prefer to peel. Ultimately, it's more important that a dish contains a large variety of fibre-rich plant-based foods than to worry too much about the preparation. I've left it completely up to you for the recipes in this book.

What about alcohol?

Although it seems that a small amount of red wine has various health benefits, it's best to keep alcohol consumption to a minimum. Perhaps just 2–3 times a week rather than every day. Real ales and ciders produced using natural fermentation methods can be drunk in moderation too. While you are following the 28-day plan, try and keep alcohol consumption low and avoid spirits, or cut out altogether, as it will help reduce your overall calories and keep you focussed. If you do decide on the occasional glass of red wine, keep the serving size small; just 125ml (an old-fashioned wine glass) is plenty. You can also use wine in cooking for adding extra flavour and depth to slow cooked stews, pasta sauces and gravies.

I'm having trouble finding unpasteurised (raw) milk cheeses in my local shops, what should I do?

Eating good quality, artisan cheeses is more important that searching out only those made with unpasteurised milk. Any soft, rinded or blue cheeses that are made by small producers are likely to contain a huge variety of beneficial microbes; those made with raw milk will simply give you a few more and heavily processed cheeses a whole lot less. Artisan cheeses are more expensive, but most cheese counters will sell portions of 25g or less, so buy just what you need. Traditionally made cheeses are more flavourful too, so a little should go a long way. Don't forget that heating the cheese will destroy the microbes, so add at the end of the cooking time, or sprinkle onto cooked dishes rather than baking if possible.

Do I need to drain and rinse canned beans?

Canned beans are cooked in the can, so potentially, the cooking liquid contains any nutrients that leach out, as well as soluble fibre that shouldn't be wasted. My rule of thumb is to buy organic beans when possible (as they don't have additives designed to improve the colour or texture of the beans), avoid beans with added salt, and use the liquid when I can. This means that I'm happy to chuck the beans and their liquid into stews and soups, but will tip into a colander and rinse off in cold water if I'm tossing through a salad or using to make bean burgers or falafel. All the recipes in this book contain canned beans, but please feel free to cook dried pulses instead if you prefer. You'll need roughly half the quantity of dried beans to get the right amount for a recipe using canned. It's well worth cooking more than you need as cooked beans will keep well in a covered container in the fridge for 2–3 days and can be successfully frozen as long as you pack into freezer bags and squeeze out as much air as possible. Simply add to cooked dishes straight from the freezer. If you are a baked bean fan, go for the reduced sugar and salt versions when you can.

When I've seen probiotic foods such as kefir and kombucha in my local health food shop, they have been really expensive. Is it essential that I include them in my diet?

It's definitely worth trying these unusual foods if you can, kefir especially has been strongly linked to a healthy gut. Making your own probiotics is simple and keeps the costs down after the initial purchases. (I found it quite a responsibility to keep everything alive and multiplying as it should, so tend not to prepare on a regular basis.) Be sure to include plenty of live yogurt in your diet, switching varieties regularly to help get the benefit of a few different bacteria, and make your own probiotic yogurt shots by blitzing live yogurt with fresh fruit. Don't forget about eating artisanal cheeses for additional probiotic benefits too.

Can I eat bread with my meals?

Yes, you can eat a high fibre wholegrain, wholemeal or sourdough bread with meals if you like. If you are trying to lose weight, I suggest keeping bread to a minimum as it tends to be high in calories and could slow down your weight loss. Half a thick slice of bread with a bowl of soup or an open sandwich topped with cooked chicken, fish or meat, plus cooked pulses, vegetables and salad should do the trick. Keep your bread in the freezer and only take out what you need. Wholegrain crispbreads are also a good choice, or brown rice cakes, for quick and easy lunches, topped with a variety of fresh veg and cheese or served with beany dips. Wholegrain flatbreads can be made into wraps – make your own or select ready-made ones with as few added ingredients as possible.

Should I choose red or ordinary brown onions, these recipes call for both?

Where possible, choose red onions as they contain more useful polyphenols and are usually a better bet when eaten raw in salads as they are a little less pungent. (The same goes for red grapes and red cabbage; choose them over the white varieties if you can.) If you don't have any red onions handy, use brown or white onions instead. Medium onions in this book are roughly 150g each, so you may need to use half for a small onion, or add extra if the recipe calls for a large onion.

I'm a real pasta lover, but I've noticed you don't include much in your meal plan. Should I avoid eating it all together?

Not at all, pasta makes a convenient and filling meal. However, if you do like to serve pasta, swap your usual kind for wholewheat pasta and cut down on the usual serving amount. Around 50g dry weight of pasta per person, cooked with lots of extra vegetables, is plenty. It's also well worth looking in the 'free-from' section of your supermarket, because that's where you'll find pastas made with beans and lentils. These types of pasta, made with legumes rather than grains, can contain up to four times as much fibre as the usual kind, and should help keep your gut microbes thriving.

Can I drink tea and coffee or diet drinks while I'm following the plan?

Yes, you can drink tea and coffee while following the plan. In fact, coffee has been shown to be good for beneficial gut bacteria. If you are aiming to lose weight, keep your intake of milky coffees low and avoid anything with added syrups or cream. Avoid diet drinks of any kind – and fizzy drinks or squash. There are all sorts of ingredients added that could disrupt your gut microbes. Stick to plain water, still or fizzy, instead. And don't forget to drink plenty of liquids while eating in this high fibre way – you'll need it to help soften your poos and keep everything moving efficiently.

What are the main points I should remember to help me achieve a healthy gut?

Overall don't stress. Don't get too bogged down on following the plan to the letter, it's more important that you learn a new, gut-healthy way of cooking and preparing meals that you actually enjoy than to worry about the finer details. Plan for a good variety of mainly plant-based foods as the focus of your meals over each day, avoid highly processed foods, reduce your meat intake and include probiotic foods where possible. Don't worry if you have the occasional blow-out but try to eat the gut-healthy way around 80 percent of the time, and especially after a course of antibiotics or an illness that has caused diarrhoea.

PART THREE

The recipes

Gut-happy platters

For several lunches during the plan, I have suggested you eat a gut-happy platter. This is a combination of easy-to-assemble ingredients, a bit like Greek meze. Eating this way means you can combine a huge variety of prebiotic, probiotic and polyphenol-rich foods easily in one meal, and gives you lots of flexibility. Gut-happy platters appear on most days of the plan each week, but you can swap them for salads or soups if you like. I find grabbing a few bits from the fridge on a busy day much more convenient than creating a recipe from scratch. You can also use any of the ingredients for a main meal salad by increasing the overall amount of vegetables and adding some leaves. If you don't feel like a hot supper one evening, gut-happy platters make a useful alternative.

You will be able to pick up most of the ingredients in the deli department of your local supermarket or delicatessen and then it won't take much to add a few cooked or raw vegetables and some salad. Mix and match the ingredients, aiming for a good selection on your plate each time.

If you go out without taking lunch and need to eat on the move, head to the deli section of a supermarket or food store. They should have enough dips, vegetable sticks, salads, fresh fruit, cooked meat and fish for you to put lunch together. You can also pick up ready-made soups and noodle dishes to reheat in the microwave at work. These foods are likely to be more processed and use more additives than your homemade version, so treat this as an occasional solution.

The platter is also a brilliant way of using up any extras that you may already have. These could include cold meats left over from a Sunday joint, or portions of baked salmon, cooked prawns, cooked and cooled rice and grains or canned beans. You can also add cooked or raw vegetables that might otherwise be wasted, small chunks of cheese and dips. Don't forget that foods such as cold cooked new potatoes, cold pasta and rice also contain resistant starch, which recent research shows helps keep your gut microbes flourishing.

Gut-happy platters:
The basics

Try to include foods from at least five of the following categories on your platter:

• Legumes, such as cooked and cooled or canned beans, lentils and peas, hummus and bean dips
• Wholegrains, including cooked grains such as bulgur wheat, barley, brown rice, wholemeal pasta or noodles, wholegrain, multi-seed, rye or wholemeal bread and flatbreads
• Prebiotic vegetables, such as artichoke hearts, asparagus, garlic, onions and leeks
• Live yogurt, yogurt cheese and yogurt-based dips
• Unpasteurised (raw milk) cheese and other cheeses
• Fruit, especially red and purple berries, red grapes, apples and bananas
• Nuts, seeds or a combination
• Cooked and cooled meat, poultry, fish and seafood
• Leaves and vegetables, including mixed salad leaves, curly endive, chicory leaves, watercress, tomatoes, peppers, radishes and beetroot, plus cold, cooked vegetables, such as roasted peppers or new potatoes.

Portion size

Although the variety and choice will make each platter feel generous, they are not about eating too much. To get the right amount, aim to cover a normal dinner plate (25cm) in a single layer, without piling up the ingredients. If you don't have room for the leaves, put them in a separate bowl and dress with a drizzle of red wine vinegar or balsamic vinegar and a slurp of extra virgin olive oil.

If weight loss is your goal, it's a good idea to have a smaller serving occasionally. Be aware that ingredients such as nuts, seeds and cheeses are high in fat. Although our bodies use the calories from foods in different ways, overeating any food will result in weight gain. A side plate with a small wedge of cheese, a bunch of grapes, a few sourdough or rye crackers, some onion relish and half an apple could be enough for a light meal. Eat mindfully and enjoy every bite.

You'll see a guideline for your platter in the photo section of this book and on my website, www.justinepattison.com.

How to assemble a gut-happy platter

- Choose a minimum of five different gut-healthy items from the list above for each platter.
- Try to have a mix of probiotic and prebiotic foods with each meal.
- Choose highly coloured vegetables and fruits.
- Mix textures and tastes on your plate to keep things interesting.
- Don't overfill your plate.

My favourite platters

To give you a few ideas, here are a few of the platters that I like to put together (they all serve one):

Mediterranean platter

- 2 tablespoons olive oil hummus
- 25g olives
- 2-3 chargrilled artichoke hearts
- 1 slice Parma ham
- 25g unpasteurised (raw milk) cheese or home-made yogurt cheese
- 2-3 roasted pepper strips
- 100g griddled courgettes and asparagus
- 20g unblanched almonds (skin on) pistachio nuts or mixed nuts
- 3 roasted garlic cloves
- 1-2 teaspoons extra virgin olive oil
- a big handful mixed leaves, including radicchio or curly endive
- 1 tsp mixed seeds

Blue cheese and fruit platter

- 25g Roquefort cheese or other unpasteurised (raw milk) cheese
- 50g red grapes
- 25g mixed nuts
- 25g cooked and cooled lentils
- 1 red chicory, thickly sliced
- 1 cooked beetroot
- 2 tablespoons full-fat live natural yogurt

Greek meze

- 25g olives
- 2 tablespoons olive oil hummus
- 2 tablespoons taramasalata or smoked mackerel dip
- 2 tablespoons baba ganoush (aubergine dip)
- 2 tablespoons minted beetroot dip
- 4 tbsp home-made tzatziki (with live yogurt)
- 25g feta cheese
- 50g red grapes
- 2 chargrilled artichoke hearts
- wholemeal flatbread (optional)

Pesto platter

- 100g assorted roasted vegetables
- 3 sun-dried tomato pieces or semi-dried tomatoes
- 50g cold, cooked wholewheat pasta
- 50g mozzarella cheese
- 1 tbsp fresh pesto sauce
- 2 tsp mixed seeds

Ploughman's lunch

- 25g unpasteurised (raw milk) cheese
- 1 slice Parma ham
- 1 pickled onion
- 25g walnuts
- 1 slice wholegrain bread
- 2 tsp onion relish or chutney
- a big handful mixed leaves, including radicchio or curly endive

Tuna and bean platter

- 80g canned tuna in water
- 50g canned mixed beans
- ½ small finely sliced red onion
- 2 tsp mixed seeds
- 25g olives
- 1 ripe tomato
- 1 tablespoon extra virgin olive oil
- a handful watercress

Smoked mackerel, beetroot and orange

- 75g smoked mackerel fillet
- 1 orange, divided into segments
- 1 cooked beetroot
- ¼ very finely sliced fennel bulb
- large handful mixed leaves
- 25g walnuts or pecan nuts
- 2 tbsp full-fat live natural yogurt
- 1 tbsp extra virgin olive oil

Asian chicken and rice

- 100g cold cooked chicken
- 50g cold cooked wholegrain rice
- 50g cold cooked edamame beans
- 100g leftover stir-fried vegetables
- 25g cashew nuts
- 2 tsp dark soy sauce
- 1 tsp toasted sesame oil

Weekend cheese platter

When you've already had a big meal at lunchtime, you may choose something lighter if you're hungry later on. This cheese platter makes a good gut-happy choice. It's also a simple lunch anytime of the week. Don't go crazy with your cheese portion. A few slender wedges of really good, unpasteurised cheese is enough. You should find that the strong flavours of artisan cheeses are far more satisfying than bland, highly processed cheese and it should contain a huge diversity of probiotic microbes too.

• 3–4 different unpasteurised (raw milk) cheeses in thin wedges (each wedge around 20g)
• 75g red grapes
• 1 apple
• 1 celery stick
• 25g mixed nuts
• 4 sourdough crackers or 1 slice dark rye bread (pumpernickel)
• Onion or plum relish (from a jar or home-made)

Unpasteurised cheeses

As discussed on page 44, current advice recommends that certain groups of people should avoid eating any soft or blue cheeses made from unpasteurized (raw) milk. These groups include very young children, the elderly, pregnant women and those whose immune system is compromised.

What to look out for

When shopping, choose items with as few added ingredients as possible and try to avoid preservatives, chemicals, emulsifiers and artificial sweeteners as they could disrupt your gut microbes. Don't worry about citric acid and acetic acid, lactic acid and ascorbic acid, which are natural preservatives used for preserving foods such as artichoke hearts and pickled onions. Pectin, which is used in some pickles and chutneys, is also fine. It's actually a prebiotic, but the amount in a dollop of chutney is modest.

You'll never be at a loss for what to have for lunch if you pick from the following lists, but feel free to add in some of your own favourites too:

Deli ingredients

- Unpasteurised (raw milk) cheeses
- Hummus (look for hummus made from olive oil)
- Full-fat live natural yogurt
- Onion dip
- Chargrilled or canned artichoke hearts
- Any green or naturally black olives, ideally packed in olive oil not brine
- Baba ganoush (aubergine dip)
- Roasted peppers
- Mushrooms à la Grecque
- Preserved garlic cloves
- Extra virgin olive oil
- Sun-dried or semi-dried tomatoes
- Tapenade
- Pickled onions
- Pickled shallots
- Grilled aubergine or courgette
- Beetroot salad

Home-cooked ingredients

- Asparagus
- Hard-boiled eggs
- New potatoes
- Wholegrain or brown rice
- Wholewheat pasta or noodles
- Soba noodles
- Bulgur wheat
- Quinoa
- Lentils
- Chickpeas
- Beans, such as red kidney beans, black beans, or cannellini beans
- Frozen peas, sweetcorn, broad beans and edamame
- Roasted vegetables
- Stir-fried vegetables

Meat, poultry and fish

- Leftover roast beef, lamb, pork, chicken, duck or turkey
- Parma ham
- Any other dry-cured ham (without preservatives except salt)
- Leftover cooked fish, such as poached salmon
- Hot and cold smoked fish, such as mackerel or salmon
- Seafood, such as cooked prawns, crab or squid
- Canned fish, such as tuna, salmon, sardines or anchovies
- Sushi

Raw vegetables and fruit

- Vegetable sticks
- Tomatoes
- Beetroot
- Radishes
- Thinly sliced asparagus
- Spring onions
- Thinly sliced red onion

- Cauliflower or broccoli florets
- Chicory leaves
- Salad leaves
- Red grapes
- Bananas
- Melon
- Tree fruits, such as apples, pears, plums, peaches or apricots
- Berries, such as strawberries, raspberries, blackcurrants, blackberries or blueberries
- Tropical fruits, such as mango, pineapple or papaya (not too much though as they contain lots of sugar)
- Citrus fruits, such as oranges, grapefruit, tangerines or clementines

Fermented foods

- Sauerkraut
- Kimchi
- Tempeh
- Kombucha
- Brine-pickled vegetables
- Kefir

Did you know...

Most supermarket versions of fermented vegetables are heat treated to destroy any harmful bacteria and give them a longer shelf life. Make your own or look for those with a label stating they contain live cultures. (See page 45 for more details.)

Breads

- Wholegrain or wholemeal
- Multi-seed
- Sourdough
- Rye bread, especially dark rye breads such as pumpernickel
- Wholewheat flatbread
- Rye or sourdough crackers

A word about bread

Supermarket bread is likely to contain sugar and a variety of chemicals, including emulsifiers and preservatives, which could affect the function of your gut microbes. These don't always appear on the label, but it's worth checking if there is one. If you can avoid this kind of bread, do – an independent bakery should be able to tell you what's in their bread, or you could make your own breads and flatbreads, which is easier than it sounds. The results should freeze really well.

Sourdough bread is made through natural fermentation and is easier to digest for some people. The same goes for breads made with ancient varieties of wheat. If you do have a problem digesting wheat-based foods, try using einkorn, spelt, emmer (farro) or khorasan (kamut) flours instead for baking. The variety will be good for you anyway.

Soups

Homemade soup is a handy way of getting lots of nutrient-and fibre-rich vegetables and pulses inside you and it makes a quick and convenient lunch or supper dish.

Most of these recipes make four servings and they all freeze really well. The preparation time can be a little long because of the vegetable peeling and chopping, but once that's done, the soup can be left to bubble away happily on the hob. I've included some dried and canned beans and lentils in a few of these soups, too, to increase the fermentable fibre. You could do the same thing to any of your favourite soup recipes. Look out for organic stock cubes or stock powder, as they won't contain artificial additives that could disrupt your gut microbes, or try swapping fresh chicken stock (recipe on page 150) for the equivalent volume of stock cubes and water.

Top your soup with a variety of fresh herbs, nuts, seeds, a drizzle of extra virgin olive oil or a generous spoonful of live yogurt or kefir to increase diversity and give it a gut-healthy boost. Why not try one or more of the following:

• Large spoonful of full-fat live natural yogurt
• Drizzle of extra virgin olive oil
• Crumbled cheese
• Finely sliced spring onions
• Garlic-infused extra virgin olive oil
• Spoonful of kimchi (see page 45)
• Olive oil croutons
• Mixed seeds or chopped mixed nuts

The recipes

Minestrone soup

Green pea and spinach soup

Hearty split pea and vegetable soup

Leek and potato soup

French onion and barley soup

Spiced lentil soup

Jerusalem artichoke soup

Chicken noodle soup

Chicken stock

HOW TO FREEZE HOMEMADE SOUP

All these soups freeze in the same way. Simply flat-freeze the cooked and cooled soup in zip-seal bags for up to four months (see page 298). Reheat the soup from frozen in a wide-based pan over a medium heat until hot throughout, stirring regularly. Add a little extra water if necessary. Alternatively, thaw in the fridge overnight and reheat in a saucepan or microwave.

Minestrone soup

A filling vegetable soup with canned beans for extra fibre. The vegetable preparation takes a little time but the soup is very quick to cook and freezes brilliantly. Serve topped with freshly grated Parmesan and basil leaves. Fresh basil pesto sauce also makes a delicious topping; either make your own (see recipe page 155) or use the chilled supermarket kind.

SERVES 4 | **PREP:** 15 MINUTES | **COOK:** 25 MINUTES

2 tbsp extra virgin olive oil
1 medium red onion, peeled and finely chopped
2 garlic cloves, peeled and finely sliced
1 medium leek, trimmed and cut into roughly 1cm slices
1 medium carrot, cut into roughly 1.5cm chunks
400g can chopped tomatoes
3 tbsp tomato purée
1 tsp mixed dried herbs

1.5 litres cold water
1 chicken or vegetable stock cube
400g can cannellini beans, drained and rinsed
1 large courgette, cut into roughly 1.5cm chunks
100g green beans, cut into roughly 2cm lengths
sea salt and black pepper
grated Parmesan and fresh basil leaves, to serve

Heat the oil in a large non-stick saucepan or sauté pan and gently fry the onion for 3 minutes, or until softened and lightly coloured, stirring often. Add the garlic, leek and carrot to the pan with the onion and stir over a low heat for 5 minutes.

Add the chopped tomatoes, tomato purée, herbs, water and stock cube and bring to the boil. Cook for 10 minutes, stirring occasionally. Add the canned beans, courgette and green beans. Return to a simmer and cook for a further 4–5 minutes or until the green vegetables are just tender, stirring regularly.

Season the soup with a little salt and lots of freshly ground black pepper. Ladle into deep bowls. Top with grated Parmesan and basil leaves.

MAKE A CHANGE

• You can also blitz all, or half of, this soup with a stick blender or a food processor until smooth.

• Use any vegetables you like to make this soup – the more variety the better! Just remember to cut dense root vegetables into small or slender pieces, so they cook quickly. Leafy greens such as shredded cabbage or kale can be added towards the end of the cooking time.

FOLLOWING THE 28-DAY PLAN?

Freeze the leftover portions of the soup to eat later in the plan. When reheating, add any leftover canned beans or vegetables to the soup.

Green pea and spinach soup

A delicious fresh-tasting soup that only takes a few minutes to knock together and makes a perfect light lunch or supper. Top with yogurt and crumbled Roquefort, goat or feta cheese if you like. A sprinkling of mixed seeds also goes well.

SERVES 4 | **PREP:** 5 MINUTES | **COOK:** 10 MINUTES

8 spring onions, trimmed and finely sliced
750g frozen peas
1.2 litres cold water
1 chicken or vegetable stock cube
15g fresh mint, leaves finely chopped (about 3 heaped tbsp), plus a few leaves to garnish

100g young spinach leaves
sea salt and black pepper
full-fat live natural yogurt, to serve (optional)

Place the onions, peas, water and stock cube in a large saucepan and bring to a simmer. Cook for 5 minutes, stirring occasionally.

Remove the pan from the heat and blitz with a stick blender until smooth. (Alternatively, cool for a few minutes then transfer in batches to a blender or food processor and blend until smooth.

Stir in the chopped mint and then the spinach leaves, a handful at a time. Warm the soup through gently for a couple of minutes without boiling. Adjust the seasoning to taste. Serve topped with spoonfuls of yogurt if you like. Garnish with a few mint leaves.

MAKE A CHANGE
This soup tastes fantastic topped with diced cooked beetroot and crumbled feta cheese. Try adding young kale leaves or other leafy greens to the soup after blitzing – it's a great way of using up mixed baby leaves or rocket from an general bag of salad.

FOLLOWING THE 28-DAY PLAN?

Freeze the leftover portions of the soup to eat later in the plan. If you transfer it to a microwavable container, it can be heated up at work. Serve with wholegrain or sourdough bread if you like.

Hearty split pea and vegetable soup

A rich and warming vegetable soup with yellow split peas. As a legume, split peas are particularly high in prebiotic fermentable fibre and will help you feel full for longer. You'll find them in most large supermarkets.

SERVES 4 | **PREP:** 15 MINUTES | **COOK:** 1–1½ HOURS

150g dried yellow split peas
2 medium onions, peeled and
   roughly chopped
4 medium carrots, roughly chopped
2 medium parsnips, roughly
   chopped
1 tbsp fresh thyme leaves
   (from 2–3 sprigs fresh thyme) or
   1½ tsp dried thyme

1 tsp ground turmeric
1.75 litres cold water
1 chicken or vegetable stock cube
sea salt and black pepper
full-fat live natural yogurt and finely
   sliced spring onions (optional),
   to serve

Put the peas, onions, carrots, parsnip, thyme, turmeric, water and stock cube in a large saucepan and bring to the boil. Reduce the heat, cover with a lid and simmer gently for 50–60 minutes or until the peas and vegetables are very soft, stirring regularly.

If the stock gets absorbed or evaporates before the peas are thoroughly cooked, add a little more water and continue simmering. Sometimes dried peas can take an extra 30–60 minutes to soften.

Remove from the heat. Blitz with a stick blender until as smooth as possible. (Alternatively, cool for a few minutes then transfer in batches to a blender or food processor and blend until smooth.)

Return to the heat and warm through gently, adding extra water if necessary until the right consistency is reached. Season to taste with salt and pepper. Serve with yogurt and garnish with finely sliced spring onions if you like.

Leek and potato soup

Heavy on prebiotic leeks, cheap and filling, this soup makes a welcome meal on a cold day and can be reheated from frozen. When the weather is hot, add a swirl of live yogurt and a sprinkling of chives for a delicious chilled Vichyssoise.

SERVES 4 | **PREP:** 10 MINUTES | **COOK:** 35 MINUTES

2 tbsp extra virgin olive oil
2 medium onions, peeled and roughly chopped
3 medium leeks (about 450g total weight), trimmed and thinly sliced, including lots of green
300g potatoes, preferably Maris Piper, peeled and cut into roughly 2cm chunks

1 litre cold water
1 chicken or vegetable stock cube
100ml semi-skimmed milk
sea salt and black pepper

Heat the oil in a large non-stick saucepan, add the onions and leeks, cover with a lid and cook over a low heat for 10 minutes, stirring occasionally until well softened.

Add the potatoes to the pan with the other vegetables and stir in the water and stock cube. Bring to the boil then reduce the heat slightly and simmer without a lid for about 20 minutes or until all the vegetables are very soft, stirring occasionally.

Remove the pan from the heat and stir in the milk. Blitz with a stick blender until smooth. (Alternatively, cool for a few minutes then transfer in batches to a blender or food processor and blend until smooth.)

Season with salt and freshly ground black pepper to taste and reheat gently, adding extra water if necessary until the right consistency is reached.

French onion and barley soup

This soup is packed with prebiotic onions and barley and is very easy to prepare – once you've got the onions sliced. I make mine with beef stock and Marmite for extra depth of flavour.

SERVES 4 | **PREP:** 15 MINUTES | **COOK:** 30–35 MINUTES

2 tbsp extra virgin olive oil
5–6 medium red onions (about 750g total weight), peeled and very thinly sliced
3 garlic cloves, peeled and crushed
1 tsp dried thyme or 1 tbsp fresh thyme leaves (from 2–3 sprigs fresh thyme), plus extra to garnish

300ml just-boiled water, plus 1 litre cold water
1 beef stock cube
1 tbsp Marmite
50g pearl barley
25g Gruyère or mature Cheddar cheese, finely grated (optional)
sea salt and black pepper

Heat the oil in a large non-stick saucepan and add the onions. Stir well then cover with a lid and cook gently for 15 minutes or until very well softened and beginning to brown, stirring occasionally. Remove the lid and add the garlic and thyme. Cook for 2 minutes more, stirring.

Pour the just-boiled water into a measuring jug and stir in the stock cube and Marmite until dissolved. Stir the barley into the cooked onions and then add the hot stock.

Top up with the cold water and bring to the boil. Reduce the heat to a simmer and cook for 25 minutes, or until the barley is tender, stirring occasionally. Season with a little salt if needed and lots of ground black pepper.

Ladle the hot soup into deep bowls and sprinkle with grated cheese and tiny sprigs of thyme if you like.

COOK'S TIP

Serve hot with toasted sourdough bread topped with grated cheese and grilled or simply topped with a little grated Parmesan or Gruyère cheese and some fresh thyme leaves.

Spiced lentil soup

This lightly curried soup is a doddle to make and provides a comforting lunch or supper on a cold day. Top with spoonfuls of yogurt and a scattering of fresh coriander.

SERVES 4 | **PREP:** 15 MINUTES | **COOK:** 30–35 MINUTES

2 tbsp extra virgin olive oil
1 medium onion, peeled and
   roughly chopped
3 medium carrots, roughly chopped
1 medium leek, trimmed and thinly
   sliced
3 garlic cloves, peeled and thinly sliced
2 sticks celery, trimmed and thinly
   sliced

1 tbsp medium curry powder
1 tsp ground turmeric
200g dried red split lentils
1.2 litres cold water
1 chicken or vegetable stock cube
sea salt and black pepper
full-fat live natural yogurt and fresh
   coriander, to serve (optional)

Heat the oil in a large non-stick saucepan and gently fry the onion for 3 minutes, stirring regularly. Add the carrots, leek, celery and garlic and cook for 2 minutes, stirring. Stir in the curry powder and turmeric and cook for a few seconds more, stirring constantly.

Tip the lentils into the pan and add the water and stock cube. Bring the liquid to the boil, then reduce the heat slightly, cover loosely with a lid and simmer gently for 20–25 minutes or until the lentils and vegetables are tender, stirring occasionally.

Remove the pan from the heat. Blitz with a stick blender until smooth. (Alternatively, cool for a few minutes then transfer in batches to a blender or food processor and blend until smooth.)

Season with salt and freshly ground black pepper to taste and reheat gently, adding extra water if necessary until the right consistency is reached. Serve topped with yogurt and freshly chopped coriander if you like.

Jerusalem artichoke soup

A warm, velvety soup that's packed with flavour and prebiotic inulin fibre. Go easy when you first try this soup – it tastes amazing but if you overdo your portion size, you will be feeling the effects for several hours. Jerusalem artichokes are known as 'fartichokes' for a reason!

SERVES 6 | **PREP:** 20 MINUTES | **COOK:** 1 HOUR

1kg Jerusalem artichokes
25g butter
1 tbsp extra virgin olive oil
1 large onion (about 250g), peeled and roughly chopped
2 garlic cloves, peeled and crushed

1.2 litres cold water
1 chicken or vegetable stock cube
fresh herbs, to garnish
150ml semi-skimmed milk
sea salt and black pepper

Peel the artichokes and put straight into a bowl of cold water to prevent them turning brown.

Melt the butter with the oil in a large non-stick saucepan and gently fry the onion for 5 minutes, or until very soft, stirring occasionally. While the onion is cooking, drain the artichokes and cut into thin slices.

Add the artichokes and garlic to the onion, cover with a loose-fitting lid and cook over a low heat for 10 minutes, stirring occasionally until the artichokes are beginning to soften.

Pour the water into the pan, and add the stock cube, a little sea salt and lots of ground black pepper. Bring the liquid to the boil, cover the pan loosely with a lid and simmer very gently for 35–40 minutes, or until the artichokes are very soft, stirring every now and then. (Add a little extra water if necessary.)

Remove the pan from the heat and stir in the milk. Blitz with a stick blender until smooth. (Alternatively, cool for a few minutes then transfer in batches to a blender or food processor and blend until smooth.) You can also pass the soup through a fine sieve to make it even more velvety.

Return the pan to the heat, and adjust the seasoning to taste. Add a little more milk or water if the soup seems to be too thick. Warm through gently, stirring regularly. Garnish with fresh herbs.

Chicken noodle soup

Chicken and vegetables in a light broth with noodles. Look out for soba noodles in your supermarket. They are usually made with a mixture of buckwheat and wholewheat flours to increase your food diversity but introduce some prebiotic fibre too.

SERVES 2 | **PREP:** 10 MINUTES | **COOK:** 15 MINUTES

1 tbsp extra virgin olive oil

1 small red onion, peeled and finely chopped

1 celery stick, trimmed and thinly sliced

1 medium carrot, cut into roughly 1cm dice

1 litre fresh chicken stock (bought or see recipe on page 150)

1 fresh bay leaf or 2 dried bay leaves

1 tsp fresh thyme leaves (from 1 sprig fresh thyme) or ½ tsp dried thyme

85g dried soba noodles (or wholewheat egg noodles)

150g cooked, skinless chicken, torn into shreds

1 small leek, trimmed and finely sliced

sea salt and black pepper

Heat the oil in a large non-stick saucepan and gently fry the onion, celery and carrot for 5 minutes or until beginning to soften, stirring occasionally. Stir the stock, bay leaf and thyme, bring to a gentle simmer and cook for 5 minutes.

While the vegetables are simmering, half fill a small pan with water and bring to the boil. Add the soba noodles, snapping in half as you place them in the pan. Stir well and return to the boil. Cook for 2 minutes, or according to the pack instructions, then drain in a sieve and add to the vegetables and stock.

Add the chicken and leek to the pan and cook for 4–5 minutes more or until the chicken is hot and the leek is tender. Season with salt and pepper.

MAKE A CHANGE

This can be made with leftover chicken from a roast or you can cook a chicken breast or a couple of thighs ready for shredding. It's best made with homemade chicken stock but chilled stock from the supermarket, although expensive, also works.

Chicken stock

A good homemade chicken stock makes a brilliant base for all types of noodle broth as well as other soups, risottos, sauces and gravy. Use the leftover carcass from a roasted chicken.

MAKES 1 LITRE | **PREP:** 15 MINUTES, PLUS STANDING | **COOK:** 1 HOUR

1 roast chicken carcass
1 medium onion, peeled and cut into chunky pieces
2 large carrots, washed well and thickly sliced
2 celery sticks, thickly sliced
2 fresh bay leaves or 3 dried bay leaves

small bunch fresh thyme or 1 tsp dried thyme
1 tsp flaked sea salt
10 black peppercorns
1.5 litres cold water

Place the chicken carcass in a large saucepan or casserole, chopping into pieces first to help it fit, if necessary. Discard any skin or fat as you go.

Put the vegetables in the pan with the chicken, tucking them in around the bones. Add the bay leaves and thyme, salt, peppercorns and water. The water shouldn't rise more than 10cm from the top of the pan, so adjust the amount you use if necessary.

Cover the pan loosely with a lid and bring to a slow simmer – the water should be bubbling extremely gently. If the water simmers or boils hard, the stock may become cloudy. Simmer very gently for 1 hour, remove from the heat and leave to stand for 30 minutes.

Carefully strain the stock, bones and vegetables through a colander into a large bowl. (Discard the bones and cooked vegetables.) Then strain the liquid through a fine sieve into a large jug. It will keep well in the fridge, covered, for up to 3 days. Scrape off the fat that solidifies on the surface before using.

FREEZING TIP
Freeze the cooked and cooled stock in small containers for up to 3 months. Reheat from frozen very gently in a saucepan over a low heat. Once thawed, bring to the boil and cook for 3 minutes.

Chicken

These chicken recipes are quick to prepare during a busy week and are easy to double up if you have more people to feed. There are a couple of gut-happy roasts for the weekend included too. By reducing the overall amount of chicken you eat, you'll find you naturally tuck into more healthy vegetables and pulses, keeping your microbes well fed and thriving. Choose organic chicken if you can. It's not cheap, but it also shouldn't contain antibiotics that could disrupt your gut microbes. And don't forget, chicken freezes very well, so tightly wrap any chicken you don't use, freeze and then thaw when you need it.

The recipes

Baked chicken breasts

Pesto chicken

Lemony chicken stir-fry

Spiced chicken with chickpeas

Cheat's chicken tikka masala

One-pan chicken tray bake

Springtime chicken

Sticky barbecue chicken

Chicken with 30 cloves of garlic

Roast chicken with savoury rice

If there is a chicken recipe in the plan that you really don't want to make, because you aren't keen on curry for instance, you can swap it for one of the other recipes on this list. Or adapt one of your favourite recipes by reducing the amount of chicken and bumping up the vegetables. Add a can of beans, lentils or barley to your casseroles too. (If you prefer using chicken thighs, adapt the recipes accordingly.)

If you are really stuck for time, bake a couple of chicken breasts and serve with at least five different vegetables and a squeeze of lemon.

Baked chicken breasts

Follow this simple method for perfectly cooked and succulent chicken breasts every time.

SERVES 2 | **PREP:** 2 minutes | **COOK:** 15 minutes

2 boneless, skinless chicken breasts (each about 150g)

2 tsp extra virgin olive oil
sea salt and black pepper

Preheat the oven to 200°C/fan oven 180°C/gas 6. Heat the oil in a medium non-stick frying pan. Season the chicken on both sides with a little salt and lots of ground black pepper.

Fry the chicken over a medium–high heat for 1–2 minutes on each side or until nicely browned. Transfer to a small baking tray and bake in the oven for 12–15 minutes, or until cooked throughout. Larger chicken breasts will take a few minutes longer. Check the chicken by slicing through the thickest part – there should be no pinkness remaining.

COOK'S TIP
When choosing chicken, try to go for the best quality you can afford. Avoid enormous chicken breasts even if they do look like great value – I've found them to be tough and chewy. Instead, select breasts that are about 150g, not much more. You'll find that free-range and organic chicken breasts tend to be smaller (and are likely to be better overall for your gut microbes).

Pesto chicken

This is a great dish that's bursting with fresh vegetables and really packs a flavour punch. Serve just as it is, or with a small serving of new potatoes or freshly cooked rice. If you don't have a food processor to make the pesto, buy a tub of good-quality fresh basil pesto sauce from the chiller department of the supermarket instead.

SERVES 2 | **PREP:** 15 minutes | **COOK:** 6–8 minutes

1 tbsp extra virgin olive oil
1 boneless, skinless chicken breast (about 150g), thinly sliced
1 medium red onion, peeled and cut into 10 wedges
1 red pepper, deseeded and cut into roughly 3cm chunks
1 medium courgette, halved lengthways and cut into roughly 1.5cm slices
½ tsp dried thyme (optional)
sea salt and black pepper

For the pesto sauce
1 tbsp pine nuts
1 garlic clove, peeled and roughly chopped
20g Parmesan cheese, cut into small chunks
15g fresh basil leaves
2 tbsp extra virgin olive oil
sea salt and black pepper

First make the pesto sauce. Put the pine nuts, garlic and Parmesan in a food processor and blitz until very finely chopped. Add the basil leaves, olive oil, a generous pinch of salt and lots of ground black pepper. Blitz to make a thick purée. You may need to remove the lid and push the mixture down a couple of times until the right consistency is reached. Set aside.

Place a large non-stick frying pan or wok over a medium–high heat. Add the 1 tablespoon of oil and when the pan is hot, add the chicken and vegetables. Sprinkle with the thyme if using. Stir-fry for 6–8 minutes, or until the chicken is thoroughly cooked and the vegetables are lightly browned. Add the pesto sauce and toss well.

MAKE A CHANGE

It's well worth making double the amount of pesto if you can, as it will keep well in a covered dish in the fridge for at least three days. If you don't have a food processor, try pounding the pine nuts, garlic, Parmesan and seasoning in a pestle and mortar until very well crushed, then transfer to a bowl and stir in finely chopped fresh basil and extra virgin olive oil. You can use pesto tossed through wholemeal pasta, as a dressing for olives, cooked and cooled new potatoes or roasted vegetables, or as a topping for grilled meats and fish. It also freezes very well.

TIME-SAVING TIP

If you buy your chicken in a double pack, you can cook the remaining breast for lunch or supper the next day.

FOLLOWING THE 28-DAY PLAN?

Serve the chicken with a small portion of new potatoes (around 100g a person) and a large mixed salad. Cook an extra 75g of potatoes per person and there will be enough for Leftover potato salad (page 273) the next day.

Lemony chicken stir-fry

This zingy stir-fry is very filling because it's jam-packed with lots of lovely vegetables, including prebiotic and fibre-rich asparagus. Serve with small portions of mixed wholegrain rice to soak up the tangy lemon sauce. Get everything ready before you start to fry, as the dish takes just 8–10 minutes to cook.

SERVES 2 | **PREP:** 15 minutes | **COOK:** 8–10 minutes

2 tbsp extra virgin olive oil
1 boneless, skinless chicken breast (about 150g), thinly sliced
1 red pepper, deseeded and cut into roughly 2.5cm chunks
1 medium carrot, thinly sliced
75g long-stemmed broccoli, trimmed and halved lengthways
75g fine asparagus, trimmed and cut in half
25g cashew nuts, roughly chopped
finely grated zest of ½ small lemon

2 large garlic cloves, peeled and very thinly sliced
1 tbsp cornflour
2 tbsp dark soy sauce
2 tbsp fresh lemon juice
150ml chicken stock (made with ½ stock cube)
4 spring onions, trimmed and cut into roughly 2cm lengths
freshly cooked wholegrain rice, to serve

Heat the oil in a large, deep non-stick frying pan or wok over a high heat and stir-fry the chicken and vegetables for 5 minutes, or until the chicken is lightly browned and the vegetables are just tender. Add the cashew nuts, lemon zest and garlic and cook for 1 minute more.

While the chicken and vegetables are frying, mix the cornflour with the soy sauce and lemon juice in a small bowl. Pour the stock into the pan and stir in the lemon juice mixture and the spring onions.

Bring to a simmer and cook for 1 or 2 minutes more or until the chicken is thoroughly cooked and sauce has thickened, stirring constantly. Serve with a small portion (around 50g dry weight per person) of freshly cooked rice.

MAKE A CHANGE

Try using tofu instead of chicken. Simply pat dry firm tofu with lots of kitchen paper after draining, then cut into cubes. Fry in the oil as above, turning occasionally until lightly browned all over, then remove from the pan before cooking the vegetables. Reheat in the sauce with the spring onions for 1–2 minutes just before serving. You can also add thawed cooked and peeled prawns instead of the chicken by adding them in the last step.

Spiced chicken with chickpeas

A chicken dish that's full of fibre thanks to its good combination of vegetables and chickpeas. Top it with generous spoonfuls of live yogurt for a decent probiotic bacteria boost and serve with a herby bulgur wheat salad for heaps of wholegrain benefits. Browning and then poaching the chicken in the rich tomato sauce guarantees it will remain tender and succulent.

SERVES 2 | **PREP:** 15 minutes | **COOK:** 30 minutes

2 small boneless, skinless chicken breasts (each about 150g)
2 tbsp extra virgin olive oil
1 medium red onion, peeled and thinly sliced
2 garlic cloves, peeled and crushed
1½ tsp ground cumin
1½ tsp ground coriander
¼–½ tsp dried chilli flakes (depending on taste)
100ml red wine or extra water
1 yellow or orange pepper, deseeded and cut into roughly 3cm chunks

400g can chopped tomatoes
120g drained and rinsed canned chickpeas (half a 400g can)
1 tbsp tomato purée
1 tsp dried mixed herbs
300ml chicken stock (made with 1 stock cube)
25g bunch fresh coriander
sea salt and black pepper
full-fat live natural yogurt and Bulgur wheat salad (page 283) or Broccoli and almond rice (page 279), to serve

Put the chicken on a board and cover with a piece of cling film. Bash the thickest part of each breast lightly with a rolling pin until the chicken is the same thickness all over. (This will help it cook evenly.) Take off the cling film and season the chicken with salt and pepper.

Heat one tablespoon of the oil in a large non-stick frying pan or sauté pan. Fry the chicken, seasoned side down, over a medium–high heat for 5 minutes until nicely browned. Turn over and season on the other side. Cook for a further 5 minutes. Transfer to a plate.

Add the onion and remaining oil to the pan and cook for 3–5 minutes, or until the onion is softened and lightly browned, stirring regularly. Stir in the garlic and spices and cook for a few seconds more. (Don't allow the garlic to burn or it will make the sauce taste bitter.)

Add the red wine or water and bubble for a few seconds before adding the pepper, canned tomatoes, chickpeas, tomato purée, mixed dried herbs and chicken stock to the pan. Reserve a few coriander sprigs for garnish and roughly chop the rest.

Add the chopped coriander to the sauce and season with lots of black pepper. Bring the sauce to the boil, then reduce the heat to a gentle simmer and cook for 5 minutes, stirring regularly.

Return the chicken breasts to the pan and simmer gently in the hot sauce without stirring for 10 minutes, or until the chicken is tender and thoroughly cooked and the sauce has thickened. Remove from the heat and scatter with the reserved coriander. Serve topped with yogurt.

FREEZING TIP
Freeze the leftover chickpeas, if using a 400g can, in a small lidded pot. Add to soups, stews and curries from frozen.

MAKE A CHANGE
• Whiz leftover chickpeas from a 400g can with a clove of garlic, 1 tbsp tahini paste, 1 tbsp fresh lemon juice, ½ tsp flaked sea salt and 3 tbsp extra virgin olive oil to make a quick hummus.
• Swap the chicken for lamb cutlets or thick fish fillets if you prefer. Poach the fish in the hot, spicy sauce for 10 minutes without pre-frying.
• For a meat-free version, fry thick aubergine slices or large Portobello mushrooms instead of the chicken until lightly browned, then simmer in the sauce as above.

Cheat's chicken tikka masala

Chicken mini breast fillets are widely available now and make this simple chicken curry even more foolproof. Look out for tikka masala paste in the world food section of your supermarket. It contains a good blend of spices, so you don't have to buy them individually. Don't leave the turmeric out as it's essential for colour and will benefit your microbes. Serve this curry with wholegrain rice, lots of probiotic live yogurt and Fresh tomato salsa (page 268).

SERVES 2 | **PREP:** 10 minutes | **COOK:** 25-30 minutes

1 tbsp extra virgin olive oil
250g chicken breast mini fillets (uncoated)
1 medium onion, peeled and finely sliced
2 garlic cloves, peeled and crushed
1 tbsp medium Indian curry paste (preferably tikka masala)
1 tsp ground turmeric
227g can chopped tomatoes
1 tbsp tomato purée

250ml chicken stock (made with ½ stock cube)
20g fresh coriander, leaves finely chopped, plus extra for garnish
1 tsp dried mixed herbs
3 tbsp live crème fraiche, double cream or full-fat live natural yogurt
sea salt and black pepper
coriander leaves and yogurt, to serve

Heat half of the oil in a medium non-stick frying pan. Season the chicken with salt and pepper. Fry the chicken over a medium–high heat for 2 minutes on each side or until lightly browned. Transfer the chicken to a plate and return the pan to the heat.

Add the remaining oil and cook the onions for 5-7 minutes, stirring regularly until very soft and just beginning to brown. Add the garlic, curry paste and turmeric and cook for another minute.

Stir in the tomatoes and add the tomato purée, chicken stock, coriander and dried mixed herbs. Bring to a simmer and cook for 10 minutes, stirring occasionally.

Return the chicken to the pan and stir in the cream or yogurt.

Simmer gently for 5 minutes or until the chicken is thoroughly cooked and the sauce is rich and thick. Adjust the seasoning to taste and garnish with fresh coriander. Serve with wholegrain rice and yogurt.

FREEZING TIP

Freeze any leftover chicken mini fillets for up to two months, wrapped tightly in a freezer bag. If you can't get hold of a small can of tomatoes for this recipe, use half a 400g can of chopped tomatoes instead and freeze what's left for up to four months or transfer to a small bowl, cover, keep in the fridge and use within three days. Use the leftover tomatoes to bulk out soups or add to bolognese, curry or stew combos.

MAKE A CHANGE

If you can't get hold of chicken mini fillets, use 2 small boneless, skinless chicken breasts instead for this recipe. Thinly slice before frying.

One-pan chicken tray bake

A beautifully simple dish of tender chicken thighs baked with lots of colourful vegetables. It's worth preparing the whole recipe even if you are cooking for one as the leftovers can be made into a salad for the next day. If you are cooking for a family, double up the ingredients and use your largest baking tray or roasting tin. Serve with a leafy salad if you like.

SERVES 2 | **PREP:** 15 minutes | **COOK:** 40 minutes

1 medium red onion, peeled and cut into 8 wedges

1 small red pepper, deseeded and cut into roughly 3cm chunks

1 small yellow or orange pepper, deseeded and cut into roughly 3cm chunks

2 large tomatoes, quartered

300g sweet potatoes, cut into roughly 3cm chunks

2 tbsp extra virgin olive oil

4 boneless, skinless chicken thighs

½ tsp smoked paprika

½ tsp dried oregano

6 unpeeled garlic cloves

½ lemon

sea salt and black pepper

Preheat the oven to 200°C/fan oven 180°C/gas 6. Put all the vegetables except the garlic in a bowl and toss with 1 tablespoon of the oil. Season with a little salt and lots of black pepper and scatter over a large baking tray.

Put the chicken thighs on a board and cut off any visible fat (kitchen scissors are good for this job). Nestle the chicken thighs amongst the vegetables, forming back into nice neat shapes. Drizzle with the remaining oil and sprinkle with the smoked paprika and oregano. Season with a little salt and pepper and roast with the vegetables for 15 minutes.

Remove the baking tray from the oven, add the garlic and turn all the vegetables. Squeeze the lemon juice over the top and return the chicken and vegetables to the oven for a further 20–25 minutes, or until the chicken is thoroughly cooked and all the vegetables are tender and lightly browned.

TIME-SAVING TIP

To help you get ahead, add a couple of extra chicken thighs to the tin (they are generally sold in packs of six anyway) and cook as above then leave to cool. Put on a plate and cover tightly. Use for salads and sandwiches. Eat within two days.

MAKE A CHANGE

Use small boneless, skinless chicken breasts for this recipe if you prefer. Add to the tin at the same time as the garlic. Drizzle with the oil and sprinkle with the oregano, paprika and seasoning before baking.

Springtime chicken

Chicken breast and colourful vegetables are cooked in a light tarragon-infused sauce. I use chicken mini fillets as they're quite cheap, are easy to cook and require no preparation. This dish goes well with a small portion of wholegrain rice or new potatoes.

SERVES 2 | **PREP:** 15 minutes | **COOK:** 15 minutes

250g boneless, skinless chicken breast mini fillets
sea salt and black pepper
15g butter
2 tsp extra virgin olive oil
1 small red onion, peeled and thinly sliced
1 garlic clove, peeled and crushed
100ml white wine
450ml chicken stock (made with 1 stock cube)
2 medium carrots, cut into roughly 1.5cm diagonal slices

5g bunch fresh tarragon (roughly 5 sprigs)
150g slender asparagus spears, trimmed and halved
1 slender leek, trimmed and cut into roughly 5mm slices
3 tbsp live crème fraiche or double cream
1 tbsp cornflour
sea salt and black pepper

Season the chicken mini fillets all over with a little flaked sea salt and plenty of freshly ground black pepper. Melt the butter with the oil in a large non-stick frying pan, sauté pan or shallow casserole and fry the chicken for 2–3 minutes on each side over a medium-high heat until lightly browned and cooked through. Transfer to a plate and set aside.

Add the onion and garlic to the pan and cook gently for 2–3 minutes, stirring frequently until the onion is softened and beginning to colour. (Take care not to let the garlic burn or it will taste bitter.) Pour the wine into the pan and let it bubble furiously for a few seconds, then stir in the stock, carrots and two of the tarragon sprigs. Cover the pan loosely with a lid or piece of foil and simmer very gently for 10 minutes, or until the carrots are just cooked.

Increase the heat and add the asparagus, leek and chicken to the pan. Cover and bring the cooking liquor to the boil and cook the green vegetables for about 3 minutes or until almost tender. While the asparagus and leeks are cooking, strip the leaves from the remaining tarragon sprigs and chop them fairly small. Mix the cornflour in a small bowl with 1 tablespoon of cold water until smooth.

Stir the cornflour mixture, crème fraiche or cream and chopped tarragon into the sauce and simmer for a further 1–2 minutes, stirring occasionally, adding a little extra water if the sauce is too thick. Season to taste and serve immediately.

MAKE A CHANGE
If you can't find chicken breast mini fillets in your local store, use one large boneless, skinless chicken breast instead. Cut into thin slices, approx 5mm thick, and cook as above.

Sticky barbecue chicken

Beautifully tender chicken thighs roasted with lots of veg and coated with a sticky barbecue-style glaze. Serve with a gut-happy salad, freshly cooked corn on the cob or canned sweetcorn and spoonfuls of full-fat live natural yogurt.

SERVES 2 | **PREP:** 15 minutes | **COOK:** 30 minutes

1 medium red onion, peeled and cut into 8 wedges

1 large red pepper, deseeded and cut into roughly 3cm chunks

1 medium courgette, halved lengthways and cut into roughly 1cm slices

300g sweet potatoes, cut into roughly 3cm chunks

2 tbsp extra virgin olive oil

4 boneless, skinless chicken thighs

½ tsp smoked paprika

sea salt and black pepper

For the barbecue-style sauce:

1 tbsp tomato purée

1 tbsp dark soy sauce

1 tbsp runny honey

1 garlic clove, peeled and crushed

Preheat the oven to 220°C/fan oven 200°C/gas 7. Put the onion, pepper, courgette and sweet potato in a bowl and toss with 1 tablespoon of the oil. Season with a little salt and lots of black pepper and scatter over a large baking tray.

Put the chicken thighs on a board and cut off any visible fat (kitchen scissors are good for this job). Nestle the chicken thighs amongst the vegetables, forming back into nice neat shapes. Drizzle the chicken with the remaining oil and sprinkle with the smoked paprika and black pepper. Season with a little salt and roast with the vegetables for 20 minutes.

While the chicken and vegetables are cooking, mix the tomato purée, soy sauce, honey and garlic together in a small bowl.

Remove the baking tray from the oven and turn all the vegetables. Brush the chicken generously with half the barbecue sauce and return to the oven for a further 5 minutes. Take out of the oven once more, brush the chicken with the remaining sauce and bake for a further 5 minutes, or until the chicken is thoroughly cooked, slightly charred and sticky. Serve with a large mixed salad and full-fat live natural yogurt.

TIME-SAVING TIP

To help you get ahead, add a couple of extra chicken thighs to the tin (they are generally sold in packs of six anyway) and cook as above then leave to cool. Put on a plate and cover tightly. Use for salads and sandwiches. Eat within two days.

MAKE A CHANGE

Use small boneless, skinless chicken breasts for this recipe if you prefer. Add to the tin with the vegetables after they have been roasting for 10 minutes, sprinkle with the seasonings and continue as above. (Chicken breasts are added to the tin later than thighs as they take less time to cook.)

Chicken with 30 cloves of garlic

This is based on the classic French recipe, but there's no need to worry that you are going to pong after eating this prebiotic-rich dish – the garlic becomes sweet and mellow during the long cooking time. I stuff my chicken with a few of the cloves to infuse it with flavour, and the rest are baked alongside the bird and are perfect for mashing into the gravy.

SERVES 4 | **PREP:** 10 minutes | **COOK:** 1¼ hours, plus standing

400g shallots (small ones, not long banana shallots)
1.5kg oven-ready fresh chicken
½ small lemon, cut in half
1 large bay leaf
30 garlic cloves (from 2–3 bulbs), unpeeled
1 tbsp extra virgin olive oil

1 tbsp fresh thyme leaves (from 2–3 sprigs fresh thyme)
150ml white wine
250ml chicken stock (made with 1 stock cube)
sea salt and black pepper

Preheat the oven to 220°C/fan oven 200°C/gas 7. Place the shallots in a heat proof bowl, cover with just-boiled water and leave to stand for 5 minutes. This will make the skins easier to remove.

Remove any trussing elastic or string from the chicken and place the lemon, bay leaf and 10 of the garlic cloves inside the cavity. Rub half the olive oil into the chicken skin then generously season the chicken with a little flaked sea salt and lots of freshly ground black pepper. Place the chicken in a medium roasting tin and sprinkle with the chopped thyme.

Drain the shallots and, once cool enough to handle, remove the skins, using a small knife to help if needed. Toss with the remaining oil then scatter around the chicken. Roast for 30 minutes.

Take the tin out of the oven and reduce the temperature to 200°C/fan oven 180°C/gas 6. Add the remaining garlic cloves to the tin and toss lightly with the shallots.

Pour the wine and chicken stock around the chicken. Cover with a large piece of kitchen foil, pinching around the edge of the tin to seal. Cook for 45–60 minutes more, or until the chicken is thoroughly cooked and the garlic is completely softened. Let the chicken rest for 15 minutes before carving into chunky pieces.

Divide amongst warmed plates and top with the baked shallots and garlic from around the chicken. Spoon over the garlicky sauce and serve with Spinach and potato mash (page 281) and assorted freshly cooked vegetables, such as green beans or asparagus and baby carrots. Squeeze the baked garlic out of its skin and mash into the potatoes.

TIME-SAVING TIP

Take any leftover chicken off the bones and discard the skin. Put on a plate, cover tightly and place in the fridge. Put the leftover shallots, garlic and cooking liquor into a bowl. Cover and place in the fridge. Reheat for lunch or supper the next day or add the cold chicken to large mixed salad.

Roast chicken with savoury rice

A super way to cook chicken and savoury rice with lots of vegetables in one pot for a quick and easy Sunday roast that should make enough leftovers for meals the next day too. Serve with a large mixed salad drizzled with a mustardy vinaigrette and you won't need any kind of gravy or sauce to accompany your bird.

SERVES 4 | **PREP:** 15 minutes | **COOK:** 1½ hours

1.5kg oven-ready fresh chicken
1 tbsp extra virgin olive oil, plus extra for greasing
sea salt and black pepper
1 medium onion, peeled and finely chopped
1 red pepper, deseeded and cut into roughly 1.5cm chunks
1 yellow pepper, deseeded and cut into roughly 1.5cm chunks
2 slender leeks, or 1 large leek, trimmed and cut into roughly 1cm slices

2 garlic cloves, peeled and very thinly sliced
½ tsp ground turmeric
1 tsp ground cumin
1 tsp ground coriander
125g easy-cook brown rice
finely grated zest and freshly squeezed juice of ½ lemon
450ml hot chicken stock (made with 1 stock cube)

Preheat the oven to 200°C/fan oven 180°C/gas 6. Lightly oil a fairly large, shallow ovenproof dish or roasting tin and place the chicken inside it. It will need to hold 2.5 litres (see tip below).

Remove the trussing elastic and retie the chicken's legs with string if you like, or leave just as they are. Season with salt and lots of ground black pepper. Roast for an hour.

Ten minutes before the chicken is ready, prepare the rice. Heat the remaining oil in a large non-stick frying pan and gently fry the onion and peppers for 5 minutes or until softened, stirring regularly. Stir in the leeks, garlic and spices and cook for 1 minute more. Add the rice and stir well.

Take the chicken out of the oven and transfer to a board. Add the rice mixture to the baking dish or tin and stir in the lemon zest and juice and hot chicken stock. Place the chicken on top and cover the whole dish with a large piece of foil, pinching around the edges to seal. Return to the oven and bake for a further 30 minutes, or until the chicken is thoroughly cooked and the rice is tender.

Carve the chicken and serve with a large mixed salad or green vegetables.

COOK'S TIPS

• Use easy-cook brown rice for this recipe. You'll sometimes find it in boil-in-the-bag packs which you need to simply snip open to use. Because it's been par-cooked and then dried, it's much quicker to cook. If you can't get hold of any, use 125g of any wholegrain rice, but boil for 15 minutes then drain before stirring into the tin; this will help give it a head-start.

• To make sure your dish or tin is large enough for this recipe, check the volume by filling with measuring jugs full of cold water. It will need to hold 2.5 litres of water – a little larger is fine, but you can't go a whole lot smaller.

FOLLOWING THE 28-DAY PLAN?

Take leftover chicken off the bones and put into a shallow dish with the rice and vegetables. Cool quickly, cover and keep in the fridge, and use within 2 days. Eat cold or reheat in a microwave until piping hot throughout.

Lamb, beef and pork

For the best gut health, it's a good idea to cut down on the amount of red meat you may be currently eating. Although it is an excellent source of protein, vitamins (including B12), iron and zinc, consuming large quantities of red meat, especially processed meats, has been strongly linked to cancer, particularly cancer of the colon (bowel cancer).

Red meat is classified as any meat that is dark red in colour before it is cooked, and includes beef, lamb and pork. Processed meat is meat that's been preserved in some way to make it stay safe to eat for longer and often has added chemicals to improve the flavour texture or odour. Processed meats include bacon, ham, sausages, salami, pepperoni and hot dogs as well as low-quality meat fillings, best avoided in ready meals or pies.

There is no need to cut red meat out altogether, unless you want to, but if you aim for a reduced number of portions a week from now on and top up with more plant-based foods instead, you are giving your gut the best chance to remain healthy and for friendly bacteria to flourish. For the purposes of the 28-day plan, I've cut red meat down to 1-2 portions a week and also limited the overall amount of red meat in every serving, which should make it easy for you to bump up your consumption of vegetables and pulses and discover a range of diverse new dishes.

The recipes

Little lamb hotpot

Quick roast lamb with mint

Lamb and sweet potato tagine

Simple lamb curry

Pan-fried pork (or chicken) with apple and leek

Steak and sweet potato wedges with blue cheese sauce

Beef and butterbean stew

Roast beef with shallots and red wine gravy

For the next 28 days, you won't be eating any processed meats preserved with chemicals, such as nitrites or nitrates. There is the opportunity to have Parma ham occasionally. I've chosen Parma ham as it is naturally dried over several months. Check the labels of any hams carefully and only select those containing nothing but the meat and salt. After the 28 days are up, only eat processed meats sparingly.

Little lamb hotpot

Hotpots are often huge but my recipe makes just enough for two and is very simple to prepare. It's also easy to double up if you want a couple of extra servings. It's probably the quickest hotpot you'll ever make and contains prebiotic onions, leeks and also pearl barley instead of potatoes.

SERVES 2 | **PREP:** 15 minutes | **COOK:** 1 hour

300g lamb neck fillet
1 tbsp extra virgin olive oil
1 medium onion, peeled and thinly sliced
1 medium leek, trimmed and cut into roughly 1cm slices
2 medium carrots, cut into roughly 1.5cm slices
50g pearl barley

400ml lamb stock (made with ½ stock cube)
1 tbsp fresh thyme leaves or ½ tsp dried thyme
1 tsp dried mint
1 tbsp Worcestershire sauce (optional)
75g frozen peas, thawed
sea salt and black pepper

Preheat the oven to 190°C/fan oven 170°C/gas 5. Trim the lamb of any hard fat that you can easily reach, and cut into roughly 4cm chunks. Season the meat generously all over with salt and pepper.

Heat the oil in a large non-stick frying pan and fry the lamb over a medium-high heat for 5 minutes, or until nicely browned on all sides. Transfer to a small flameproof casserole.

Add the onions to the frying pan and cook for 3 minutes, stirring. Add the leeks and carrots and cook together for 2 minutes more, stirring constantly. Add to the lamb and stir in the pearl barley, stock, thyme, mint and Worcestershire sauce, if using. Season well with a little salt and lots of ground black pepper.

Bring to a simmer then cover with a lid and transfer carefully to the oven. Cook for 45–55 minutes, or until the lamb and pearl barley are tender. Take out of the oven, add the peas then cover and return to the oven for a further 3 minutes. Adjust the seasoning to taste before serving in warmed bowls.

FREEZING TIP

Freeze the cooked and cooled hotpot in zip-seal bags or freezer-proof containers for up to three months. Thaw overnight in the fridge then reheat in the microwave or a wide-based saucepan with an extra 100ml water, stirring occasionally until piping hot.

TIME-SAVING TIP

If you want to make extra hotpot for the freezer, double up on all the ingredients but reduce the stock to 700ml. Fry the lamb in two batches before adding to the casserole.

Quick roast lamb with mint

Look out for extra-trimmed racks of lamb for this recipe as
all the hard work will have been done for you. Rack of lamb
is fairly pricy, so this is the perfect dish to save for a weekend
lunch. It's easy to double up for four and is ready to serve in
under an hour.

SERVES 2 | **PREP:** 15 minutes | **COOK:** 40 minutes

1 rack of lamb, extra trimmed
   (roughly 300g)
1 tbsp extra virgin olive oil
150g carrots cut into roughly 1.5cm
   wide batons
225g baby new potatoes, halved
1 medium courgette, trimmed and
   cut into roughly 1.5cm slices
100g asparagus, trimmed and
   snapped in half

100g frozen peas
sea salt and black pepper

For the fresh mint sauce:
15g bunch fresh mint
1 tbsp caster sugar
1 tsp red wine vinegar
3 tbsp extra virgin olive oil
sea salt and black pepper

Preheat oven to 200°C/fan oven 180°C /gas 6. Season the lamb
all over with a little salt and plenty of freshly ground black pepper.
Pour 1 teaspoon of the oil into a non-stick frying pan and place
over a medium–high heat.

Cook the lamb for 2–3 minutes, turning the rack after each
minute to ensure every side of the lamb has lightly browned.
Set aside.

Place the carrots and potatoes in a small roasting tin and drizzle
with the remaining oil. Toss well together. Season with salt and lots
of freshly ground black pepper. Roast for 15 minutes.

While the potatoes and carrots are roasting, make the mint
sauce: strip the leaves from the mint and finely chop. Put in a small
bowl and stir in the sugar and vinegar. Slowly whisk in the olive oil
and then season to taste with salt and pepper.

Take the carrots and potatoes out of the oven and turn with a
spatula. Add the courgettes and toss together. Transfer the lamb
to the same tin and roast in the oven for 20 minutes, adding the
asparagus for the last 10 minutes of the cooking time.

Take the roasting tin out of the oven and place the lamb on a board. Cover loosely with foil and leave to rest for 5 minutes. Scatter the peas into the pan with the other vegetables and toss lightly. Return to the oven for 5 minutes or until all the vegetables are tender.

Carve the lamb into individual cutlets. Divide the vegetables between 2 warmed plates and top with the lamb. Season with a little salt and pepper and spoon over the mint sauce to serve.

COOK'S TIP
Cut the asparagus roughly halfway down the stem after trimming. If you can only get hold of thicker, older asparagus, cut in half lengthways too.

TIME-SAVING TIP
Add a few extra vegetables to the pan and eat leftovers for lunch the next day.

MAKE A CHANGE
If you don't fancy lamb, make this dish with chicken breasts or thighs instead. Serve with fresh pesto sauce instead of mint sauce if you like.

Lamb and sweet potato tagine

This recipe is based on one of my favourite lamb tagine recipes. It makes generous portions, so you can always save some for lunch the next day. It uses ras-el-hanout spice mix and harissa paste, which are available in larger supermarkets. Both will last for ages in the store cupboard and fridge.

Serve with a large mixed salad and small portions of bulgur wheat or rice and lots of full-fat live natural yogurt.

SERVES 2 | **PREP:** 15 minutes | **COOK:** 55 minutes

300g lamb neck fillet
1 tbsp extra virgin olive oil
1 medium onion, peeled and thinly sliced
2 garlic cloves, peeled and crushed
1 tbsp ras-el-hanout spice mix
1 tsp cumin seeds
1 tsp ground turmeric
150g sweet potatoes, cut into roughly 3cm chunks
120g canned chickpeas (½ a 400g can), drained and rinsed
400g can chopped tomatoes
50g dried apricots, halved (optional)
300ml lamb stock (made with ½ stock cube)
2 tsp harissa paste (from a jar)
1 tbsp runny honey
20g bunch of fresh coriander, plus extra to garnish
sea salt and black pepper
full-fat live natural yogurt, to serve

Preheat the oven to 190°C/fan oven 170°C/gas 5. Trim the lamb neck fillet of any hard fat that you can easily reach, and cut the lamb into roughly 4cm chunks. Season all over with salt and pepper.

Heat the oil in a large non-stick frying pan and fry the lamb and onions for 5 minutes or until the lamb is lightly browned and the onions are softened, stirring regularly. Stir in the garlic, ras-el-hanout, cumin seeds and turmeric and cook for a few seconds more.

Tip into a small flameproof casserole and add the sweet potatoes, chickpeas, tomatoes, apricots (if using), lamb stock, harissa paste and honey. Season with lots of ground black pepper. Finely chop the coriander leaves and stalks and stir into the lamb and vegetables.

Bring to a simmer on the hob then cover with a lid and transfer carefully to the oven. Cook for 45–55 minutes, or until the lamb and vegetables are tender and the sauce is thick and aromatic. Scatter with the reserved coriander and serve with freshly cooked bulgur wheat and lots of yogurt.

FREEZING TIP
• Freeze the cooked and cooled tagine in zip-seal bags or freezer-proof containers for up to two months. Thaw overnight in the fridge then reheat in the microwave or a wide-based saucepan with an extra 100ml water, stirring occasionally until piping hot.
• Use the leftover chickpeas from a 400g can in salads, stews and curries. You can freeze in small bags, tightly wrapped, for up to one month.

MAKE A CHANGE
If you can't find ras-el-hanout in your local store, use 1½ tsp ground coriander, 1 tsp ground cumin and ½ tsp ground paprika instead.

Simple lamb curry

A rich-tasting curry with tender lamb and prebiotic onions and lentils. I've used lamb neck fillet as it stays more tender than leg and is much easier to prepare than shoulder, but you could use cutlets or chops instead. Serve with small portions of freshly cooked wholegrain rice, topped with yogurt, cucumber and mint. Freeze any leftovers for another day.

SERVES 4 | **PREP:** 20 minutes | **COOK:** 1 hour–1¼ hours

600g lamb neck fillets
2 tbsp extra virgin olive oil
2 medium onions, peeled and finely sliced
150g button mushrooms, halved
2 garlic cloves, peeled and crushed
25g chunk fresh root ginger, peeled and finely grated
3 tbsp medium Indian curry paste (such as tikka masala)

1 tsp ground turmeric
400g can chopped tomatoes
150g dried red split lentils
1 tsp caster sugar
bunch fresh coriander, roughly chopped, including the stalks
500ml lamb stock (made with 1 stock cube)
100g young spinach leaves
sea salt and black pepper

Preheat the oven to 200°C/fan oven 180°C/gas 6. Trim the lamb neck of any hard fat that you can easily reach and cut into roughly 4cm chunks. Season with salt and lots of black pepper.

Heat 1 tablespoon of the oil in a large non-stick frying pan and fry the lamb in two batches over a medium–high heat until browned on all sides. Transfer to a medium flameproof casserole and return the frying pan to the heat.

Add the remaining oil and fry the onions and mushrooms for 5–6 minutes, or until softened and lightly browned, stirring regularly. Add the garlic, ginger, curry paste and turmeric to the onions and cook for 1 minute more, stirring constantly.

Add to the lamb and stir in the tomatoes, lentils, caster sugar and coriander. Pour over the stock, stir well and cover with a lid. Bring to a simmer, then transfer carefully to the oven and cook for 45–55 minutes, or until the lamb is tender and the sauce is thick.

Take the dish out of the oven and stir in the spinach leaves, a handful at a time, adding a splash of just boiled water if necessary.

Add a little more salt and pepper to taste. Serve with small portions of brown basmati or wholegrain rice and lots of full-fat live natural yogurt, garnished with extra coriander.

FREEZING TIP

Freeze the cooled curry in zip-seal bags or in foil containers for up to three months. Thaw in the fridge overnight. Reheat thoroughly in the microwave or a large, wide-based saucepan with an extra 100ml water, stirring occasionally until piping hot throughout.

MAKE A CHANGE

Swap the lamb for 6–8 skinless, boneless chicken thighs if you like. Simply trim off any fat and cut each thigh into 3 chunks. To make it meat-free, use medium aubergines, cut into roughly 3cm chunks, instead of the lamb and fry with 2–3 tbsp extra oil.

Pan-fried pork (or chicken) with apple and leek

This quick midweek supper is made with lean pork steaks – try to buy free-range if you can – in a tangy sauce made from prebiotic onion, leek and apple. It goes well with shredded Savoy cabbage or kale and carrots. If you aren't keen on pork, make it with chicken breast instead.

SERVES 2 | **PREP:** 10 minutes | **COOK:** 15 minutes

1 medium red-skinned eating apple

2 pork loin steaks

15g butter

1 tbsp extra virgin olive oil

1 medium red onion, peeled and thinly sliced

1 slender leek, trimmed and cut into roughly 5mm slices

2 garlic cloves, peeled and crushed

250ml cider or apple juice

1 tbsp runny honey

3 fresh sage leaves, thinly sliced, plus extra to garnish (optional)

2 tsp cornflour

1 tbsp cold water

3 tbsp half fat live crème fraiche (optional)

sea salt and black pepper

Cut the apple into quarters and remove the core. Slice thickly and put to one side. Season the pork with a little salt and lots of ground black pepper.

Melt the butter in a large non-stick frying pan over a high heat. Fry the apple slices for 1–2 minutes on each side until golden brown, then transfer to a plate.

Pour 1 tablespoon of the oil into the pan and fry the pork over a medium–high heat for about 3 minutes on each side or until nicely browned and just cooked. Transfer the pork to a separate plate.

Tip the onion and leek into the same frying pan and cook over a medium heat for 4–5 minutes or until softened, stirring occasionally. Add the garlic and cook for a few seconds more.

Stir in the cider or apple juice, honey and sage leaves, if using. Season with salt and pepper. Bring the liquid to the boil and cook for 3 minutes, stirring occasionally.

Mix the cornflour with the cold water in a small bowl until smooth. Stir into the cider sauce and cook for around 30 seconds, stirring constantly until smooth. Add the crème fraiche, if using, and adjust the seasoning to taste. Return the pork and apples to the pan and cook in the bubbling sauce for 3 minutes or until hot throughout, stirring occasionally. Serve with lots of freshly cooked vegetables.

MAKE A CHANGE
Instead of the pork, thinly slice (approx 5mm) 1 large boneless, skinless chicken breast and stir-fry in the oil until lightly browned. Transfer to a plate while the sauce is made, then return to the pan in the last step and reheat for 2–3 minutes, or until hot throughout.

FOLLOWING THE 28-DAY PLAN?

If you are following the plan and not doubling up the recipe, you will end up with cider or apple juice leftover. The good news is that it can be frozen in small lidded containers for up to 3 months.

Steak and sweet potato wedges with blue cheese sauce

Lean sirloin steak is seasoned with black pepper and pan-fried or griddled then served with a microbe-boosting blue cheese sauce and sweet potato wedges. Serve with my Simple gut-happy salad (page 271).

SERVES 2 | **PREP:** 15 minutes | **COOK:** 35 minutes

350g sweet potatoes
2 tbsp extra virgin olive oil
1 tsp coarsely ground black pepper, plus extra to season
flaked sea salt
2 x 150g sirloin, fillet or rump steak
Simple gut-happy salad, to serve (page 271)

For the blue cheese sauce:
25g Roquefort cheese, or other blue cheese, rind removed
3 tbsp full-fat live natural yogurt
½ tsp red wine vinegar
1 tbsp extra virgin olive oil

Preheat the oven to 220°C/fan oven 200°C/gas 7. Peel the sweet potatoes and cut into long wedges, around 2.5cm wide. Half fill a medium saucepan with water and bring to the boil.

Add the sweet potato wedges and return to the boil. Cook for 4 minutes then drain and return to the saucepan. Pour over 1 tablespoon of the oil and season with a little salt and lots of ground black pepper. Toss until the potatoes are lightly coated with the oil.

Scatter the wedges over a baking tray and cook in the oven for 15 minutes, then turn with a spatula and cook for a further 10 minutes or until tender and golden.

While the potatoes are cooking, heat the oil in a large non-stick frying pan over a medium–high heat. Season the steak all over with the 1 teaspoon of coarsely ground pepper and cook for 2–4 minutes on each side or until done to taste. The thicker the steak, the longer it will take to cook. Divide between 2 warmed plates and leave to rest for just 5 minutes.

Mix together the cheese and yogurt in a small bowl using a fork. Stir in the vinegar until well combined then add the oil and combine well. Season to taste with ground black pepper. Pour into 2 tiny dishes.

Divide the wedges between the 2 plates and place a pot of sauce on each one. Serve with a simple gut-happy salad. (Don't pour the sauce over the steak or it will cool it.)

COOK'S TIP
Why not serve a baked tomato alongside the steak and wedges? Simply cut a large tomato in half and season with a little salt and black pepper. Place on the same baking tray as the sweet potatoes for the last 10 minutes of their cooking time.

Beef and butterbean stew

One of my all-time favourite stews, the tender beef, tomatoes and fibre-rich butterbeans go brilliantly together and make a warming meal that's perfect for a cold winter's day.

SERVES 4 | **PREP:** 10 minutes | **COOK:** 2 hours

600g good-quality braising beef (ideally chuck steak), trimmed of hard fat and cut into roughly 3cm chunks
2 tbsp extra virgin olive oil
2 medium onions, peeled and thinly sliced
2 sticks celery, thinly sliced
2 garlic cloves, peeled and crushed
400g can chopped tomatoes
2 tbsp tomato purée
300ml beef stock (made with 1 stock cube)
1 tsp dried mixed herbs
1 fresh bay leaf or 2 dried bay leaves
2 medium carrots, cut into roughly 2cm diagonal slices
400g can butterbeans
sea salt and black pepper

Preheat the oven to 180°C/fan oven 160°C/gas 4. Season the beef all over with salt and pepper. Heat half the oil in a large non-stick frying pan and fry the beef in two batches for 3–4 minutes or until nicely browned all over. Transfer to a flameproof casserole.

Return the pan to the heat and add the remaining oil. Gently fry the onions and celery for 5 minutes, or until softened and lightly browned, stirring occasionally. Add the garlic and cook for a few seconds more, stirring. Add to the beef and stir in the tomatoes, tomato purée, beef stock and herbs. Bring the liquid to a simmer, then cover and transfer carefully to the oven. Cook for 1 hour.

Take the pan out of the oven and stir in the carrots and beans. Return to the oven for a further hour, or until the beef is beautifully tender and the sauce has thickened. Adjust the seasoning to taste before serving.

FREEZING TIP
Freeze any leftover cooked and cooled stew in labelled zip-seal bags for up to three months. Thaw overnight in the fridge then reheat in the microwave or a wide-based saucepan over a medium heat, stirring regularly until piping hot throughout.

Roast beef with shallots and red wine gravy

Roast beef makes a welcome Sunday lunch and if you cook a larger joint than you need, you'll have plenty left over for a salad the next day. The shallots and red wine gravy will help keep your microbes happy, but don't forget to serve with a wide selection of different vegetables too. I prefer to use sirloin or rolled rib for roasting but a good-quality piece of topside is almost as good, especially when cooked rare.

SERVES 6 | **PREP:** 10 minutes | **COOK:** 1 hour

1kg beef topside, sirloin or boned and rolled rib
4 large long shallots or small onions, peeled and quartered
1 tbsp extra virgin olive oil
100ml red wine

400ml beef stock (made with 1 stock cube)
1 tsp tomato purée
4 tsp cornflour
2 tbsp cold water
sea salt and black pepper

Preheat the oven to 200°C/fan oven 180°C/gas 6. Season the beef on all sides with salt and plenty of freshly ground black pepper. Brush a large non-stick frying pan with a little of the oil and place over a medium–high heat. Add the beef to the pan and brown for 8–10 minutes, turning every now and again.

Put the beef in a sturdy roasting tin and roast for 45 minutes. Add 10 minutes to the cooking time for medium and 20 minutes for well-done beef. Toss the shallots or onions with the remaining oil. Add the shallots or onions to the pan with the beef for the last 30 minutes of the beef cooking time, scattering around the meat.

Remove the tin from the oven and transfer the beef to a board. Loosely cover with foil and leave to rest for 15 minutes. Place the roasting tin containing the shallots on the hob, add the red wine, then the beef stock and tomato purée and bring to a simmer. Stir to lift the tasty juices from the bottom of the pan. Mix the cornflour with the water until smooth and stir into the tin.

Return to a simmer and cook for 5 minutes, stirring constantly.

Season to taste with plenty of freshly ground black pepper – lots more than you might think you would need.

Carve the beef into thin slices and tip any of the carving and resting juices into the gravy. Put the beef on 4 warmed plates and serve with the shallot gravy. Spinach or celeriac mash and lots of freshly cooked vegetables also go well.

FREEZING TIP
Freeze any leftover beef from a large joint or save it in the fridge for a salad for lunch the next day. If freezing, put the beef into freeze-proof containers and cover with gravy to keep moist. Thaw overnight in the fridge then reheat in the microwave or a large non-stick frying pan. It won't be rare when you eat it second time around, but it's still a useful meal to have on standby.

COOK'S TIP
Sirloin and rolled rib tend to be evenly sized from one end to the other but topside and top rump (which you can also use) vary widely. It's sometimes difficult to tell when they are in the pack as the size is distorted. If you do end up buying a piece that is far narrower at one end, or almost triangular, you'll need to adjust the cooking times above. You will probably find that the beef needs just 30–40 minutes to be cooked rare, so leave the shallots and onions in a bit longer to finish cooking while the meat is resting. Invest in a digital food thermometer if you can – they are an amazing bit of kitchen kit and a huge help for foolproof meat cooking.

MAKE A CHANGE
If you don't fancy beef, cook a boned and tied loin of pork or lamb leg instead and adjust the cooking times accordingly. Switch the stock cube to a complementary flavour too.

Fish and seafood

If you don't already cook fish on a regular basis, it's worth making a special effort to incorporate more into your diet. Fish is packed with protein and fatty fish, such as salmon and mackerel, contain oils like omega-3, that research has shown could help good gut bacteria flourish and prevent weight gain, when compared to eating saturated fats such as those found in meat.

I've selected quick and easy recipes that even the least-experienced fish cook should cope with very easily. When shopping, try and buy wild fish and seafood if possible. Fish and prawn farms use lots of antibiotics to keep the fish healthy and, as with meat, small amounts can then be consumed by us, potentially causing disruption to our gut microbes. Eating a diverse diet, full of prebiotic and probiotic foods, should help our microbes to counteract this but it's best to be on the safe side and avoid farmed fish where possible.

The recipes

Sea bass and roasted vegetables

Sea bass fillets are quick and easy to cook. For this recipe, a selection of Mediterranean-style vegetables are roasted with a little chilli and when almost cooked, the fish is nestled amongst them and returned to the oven for just 10 minutes more.

SERVES 2 | **PREP:** 15 minutes | **COOK:** 40 minutes

1 red pepper, deseeded and cut into roughly 2cm chunks

1 yellow or orange pepper, deseeded and cut into roughly 2cm chunks

1 medium sweet potato (about 300g), cut into roughly 2cm chunks

2 medium courgettes, cut in half lengthways and then into roughly 1.5cm slices

1 medium red onion, peeled and cut into 10 thin wedges

2 tbsp extra virgin olive oil, plus extra for drizzling

½ tsp dried chilli flakes (optional)

4 sun-dried tomato pieces (from a jar), drained and sliced

3 tbsp pine nuts

2 sea bass, bream or mackerel fillets, each about 125g

handful small fresh basil leaves (optional)

½ lemon, sliced

sea salt and black pepper

Preheat the oven to 220°C/fan oven 200°C/gas 7. Put all the vegetables in a large bowl and toss with the oil. Season with a large pinch of salt and lots of ground black pepper. Scatter over a baking tray in a single layer and roast for 30 minutes.

Take the baking tray out of the oven and sprinkle the chilli flakes, if using, sun-dried tomatoes and pine nuts over the vegetables. Turn the vegetables, mixing with the added ingredients, and push to one side of the tin. Place the fish fillets on the tray in the space left by the vegetables. Season and top with 4 slices of lemon. Return to the oven for 10–15 minutes or until the fish is cooked through and the vegetables are softened and lightly browned.

Divide between 2 plates and drizzle with a little more oil, scatter with basil leaves and serve.

Simple soy and ginger salmon

This is the sort of dish that I go back to time and time again. It only contains a few simple ingredients and is a doddle to knock together. It's worth doubling up the salmon and glaze for this recipe, as it's also wonderful eaten cold with salad for a quick and easy lunch the next day. I often serve it with my Simple vegetable stir-fry (page 282).

SERVES 2 | **PREP:** 10 minutes | **COOK:** 20 minutes

20g chunk fresh root ginger
1 tbsp dark soy sauce
1 tbsp runny honey
1 garlic clove, peeled and crushed
¼–½ tsp dried chilli flakes, depending on taste

2 salmon fillets, each about 125g
2 spring onions
sea salt and ground black pepper
Simple vegetable stir-fry (page 195), to serve

Preheat the oven to 200°C/fan oven 180°C/gas 6 and line a small, shallow ovenproof dish, baking tray or roasting tin with a piece of kitchen foil.

Peel the ginger and thinly slice. Pile the ginger slices up into small stacks of 4–5 slices and cut into very fine matchsticks. Put into a medium bowl. Add to the soy sauce, honey, garlic and chilli flakes, if using, and mix well together. Add the salmon and turn to coat fully in the sauce. (If you have time, you can cover the dish and marinate the salmon in the fridge for 30 minutes or up to eight hours before cooking.)

Put the salmon fillets in the prepared dish or tin, skin-side down, and spoon over the soy sauce mixture. Trim and cut the spring onions into roughly 2cm lengths. Sprinkle them over the salmon and season with salt and pepper. Bake the salmon for 15 minutes or until just cooked through.

Place the salmon on 2 plates, discarding the skin. Spoon the spring onions and hot cooking liquor over the fish and serve with stir-fried vegetables and a small portion of rice or noodles.

Cook 80g wholegrain rice and 50g puy or green lentils in boiling water until tender. Serve half with the salmon - tossed with freshly chopped parsley if you like - and save half to go into a salad the next day. Cool the reserved portions quickly by rinsing in a sieve under cold water once the hot rice has been served. Keep in a covered container in the fridge and eat within two days. Cook 1-2 extra salmon fillets in the same pan as above, but transfer to a plate once ready. Cool then cover and chill.

One-pan baked fish

You can use any thick fish fillet you like for this simple recipe – think about trying a different fish each time you make it. Even fish fillets, such as sea bass or bream, can be used. If picking salmon, it's worth adding a couple of extra pieces of fish to the tin as the cold salmon makes a great base for a gut-happy platter or salad for the next day.

SERVES 2 | **PREP:** 15 minutes | **COOK:** 30 minutes

1 small red onion, peeled and cut into 12 wedges

1 small red pepper, deseeded and cut into roughly 3cm chunks

1 small yellow or orange pepper, deseeded and cut into roughly 3cm chunks

1 medium courgette, cut into roughly 1.5cm slices

1 tbsp extra virgin olive oil, plus extra for drizzling

2 thick fish fillets, such as salmon, cod or haddock, each about 125g

200g cherry tomatoes

handful fresh basil leaves, roughly torn

sea salt and black pepper

Preheat the oven to 220°C/fan oven 200°C/gas 7. Put the onion, peppers and courgette in a large roasting tin, drizzle over the oil and season with salt and pepper. Toss lightly together then bake for 15 minutes.

Take the tin out of the oven and turn the vegetables. Make 2 spaces and nestle the fish into the tray, skin-side down. Add the cherry tomatoes and season with black pepper.

Bake for a further 12–15 minutes or until the fish is just cooked and the vegetables are tender and lightly charred. Drizzle with a little extra olive oil. Scatter the basil leaves over just before serving.

MAKE A CHANGE
Throw a few olives into the tin at the same time as the salmon for an extra polyphenol boost. Cherry tomatoes can be cooked on the vine with the fish; simply snip into short lengths, each holding 4–5 tomatoes.

Baked fish with fennel and smashed potatoes

This simple recipe roasts fish in a tray with fennel, crispy potatoes and juicy tomatoes. It can be made with any fresh fish fillets you like – just bear in mind that the thicker they are, the longer they will take to cook. Thin fillets, such as mackerel, bream and sea bass will take around 10–12 minutes and thicker salmon or cod fillets could take up to 15 minutes. Add freshly boiled seasonal vegetables to complete your meal – runner beans, asparagus, carrots and leeks go particularly well.

SERVES 2 | **PREP:** 10 minutes | **COOK:** 45 minutes

250g baby new potatoes, halved if large

½ fennel bulb, very thinly sliced from root to top

2½ tbsp extra virgin olive oil

3 spring onions, trimmed and finely sliced

150g cherry tomatoes, cut in half

50g olives, any colour, drained (optional)

2 sea bream or mackerel fillets, each about 125g

finely grated zest of ¼ lemon

1 tsp fresh thyme leaves

2 lemon wedges, for squeezing

sea salt and black pepper

Preheat the oven to 220°C/fan oven 200°C/gas 7. Put the potatoes in a medium saucepan and cover with cold water. Place over a high heat and bring to the boil. Cook for 10 minutes then take off the heat and drain well in a colander. The potatoes should be not quite soft.

Tip the potatoes onto a large baking tray and very lightly crush with a fork then push to one side. Add the sliced fennel to the tray, season both vegetables with a little salt and plenty of ground black pepper. Drizzle with 2 tablespoons of the oil. Bake for 15 minutes, or until the potatoes are getting crusty around the edges.

Take the potatoes out of the oven and scatter over the spring onions, tomatoes and olives, if using. Toss together lightly. Make 2 gaps in the vegetables and place the fish fillets on the baking tray, skin-side up. Drizzle the fish with the remaining oil. Mix the lemon zest and thyme leaves together and sprinkle over the fish fillets.

Return the tray to the oven for a further 10–15 minutes, or until the fish is cooked and the tomatoes have softened. Serve with freshly cooked vegetables and lemon wedges for squeezing.

Zingy Asian cod

Plainly cooked fish can sometimes be a little dull but not this time – my zingy Asian-inspired dressing really brings it to life. Serve with small portions of wholegrain rice, wholewheat noodles or soba noodles if you like.

SERVES 2 | **PREP:** 5 minutes | **COOK:** 10 minutes

2 tsp extra virgin olive oil
2 thick white fish fillets (such as cod or haddock) with skin, each about 150g
sea salt and black pepper
100g fine asparagus or mangetout, trimmed
100g long-stemmed broccoli, trimmed and cut in half lengthways

1 medium leek, trimmed and cut into roughly 1cm slices
lime wedges, for squeezing

For the lime dressing:
1 tbsp fresh lime juice
1 tsp Thai fish sauce (nam pla)
1 tbsp soft light brown sugar
¼ tsp dried chilli flakes

To make the dressing, mix the lime juice, fish sauce, brown sugar and chilli and set aside. Fill a large saucepan pan a third of the way with water and bring it to the boil.

Heat 2 teaspoons of the oil in a medium non-stick frying pan and place over a high heat. Season the fish all over with salt and pepper. Cook the fish, skin-side down, for 3 minutes or until the skin is crisp.

Turn the fish over, reduce the heat to low and cook for a further 3–5 minutes until just cooked, depending on thickness. The centre will be creamy white rather than translucent when it is cooked.

While the fish is cooking, add the vegetables to the boiling water, return to the boil and cook for 2 minutes or until just tender. Drain in a colander and divide between 2 warmed plates.

Top the vegetables with the fish and spoon over the dressing. Serve with lime wedges for squeezing.

Italian fish stew

A warming, rich vegetable and fish stew with bags of bold Mediterranean flavour. I love to serve it with warm garlicky beans and a colourful mixed salad. It's also brilliant topped with a little of my yogurt mayonnaise.

SERVES 2 | **PREP:** 15 minutes | **COOK:** 20 minutes

2 tbsp extra virgin olive oil
1 small red onion, peeled and thinly sliced
½ small fennel bulb (about 150g), trimmed and thinly sliced
1 medium courgette, halved lengthways and cut into roughly 1.5cm slices
2 garlic cloves, peeled and thinly sliced
¼-½ tsp dried chilli flakes (depending on taste)
1 tsp ground coriander
1 tsp dried oregano
2 tbsp tomato purée
100ml red wine

400g can chopped cherry tomatoes or chopped tomatoes
50g black olives, preferably Kalamata, drained (and pitted if preferred)
1 tsp caster sugar
200g thick, skinless white fish fillet (such as cod or haddock), cut into roughly 4cm chunks
sea salt and black pepper
fresh chopped parsley and extra virgin olive oil, to garnish (optional)
Warm beans with garlic and lemon (page 284) and Yogurt mayonnaise (page 294) to serve

Heat the oil in a large non-stick frying pan or sauté pan and gently fry the onion and fennel for 5 minutes or until well softened, stirring regularly. Add the courgette and cook for 3 minutes more, stirring.

Add the garlic, chilli, coriander and oregano and cook for a few seconds more. Stir in the tomato purée and wine. Bring to a simmer and cook for 1 minute, stirring. Add the canned tomatoes, olives and sugar and cook for 3 minutes, stirring constantly. Season to taste with salt and pepper.

Add the fish pieces and simmer gently for 5-6 minutes, or until just cooked and beginning to flake. (The time will depend on the thickness of your fish pieces.) Stir occasionally and gently, taking care not to break up the fish.

Scatter parsley over the top if using and drizzle with a little more olive oil to serve. (Watch out for olive stones when eating if using the unpitted type.)

FREEZING TIP
Flat-freeze this sauce for up to three months, if made in advance. Reheat from frozen in a large wide-based pan with an extra 100ml water until hot, then add fresh fish pieces and continue cooking as above.

MAKE A CHANGE
The slight aniseed taste of the fennel goes particularly well with fish but if you can't get hold of any, use cubes of yellow pepper or aubergine instead.

Thai fish curry

A really simple and quick supper dish with onion, garlic and antioxidant-rich peppers. It's a great introduction to cooking and eating fish if you're a bit of a novice and seems to go down well with everyone. Serve with Broccoli and almond rice (page 279) for an extra wholegrain and vitamin boost.

SERVES 2 | **PREP:** 15 minutes | **COOK:** 12 minutes

50g block coconut cream
250ml just-boiled water
2 tbsp extra virgin olive oil
1 medium red onion, peeled and cut into thin wedges
1 red pepper, deseeded and cut into roughly 3cm chunks
1 yellow or orange pepper, deseeded and cut into roughly 3cm chunks
2 garlic cloves, peeled and very thinly sliced
2 tbsp Thai red curry paste (from a jar)

4 kaffir lime leaves, preferably fresh
1 tbsp nam pla (Thai fish sauce)
2 tsp soft light brown sugar or runny honey
1 tsp cornflour mixed with 2 tsp cold water to form smooth paste
200g fresh, skinless thick white fish fillet (such as haddock or cod), cut into roughly 3cm chunks
fresh coriander, to garnish (optional)
Broccoli and almond rice (page 279), to serve

Put the coconut cream into a heatproof bowl and add the just-boiled water. Stir until the coconut dissolves. Don't expect it to be completely smooth; it will remain slightly grainy.

Heat the oil in a large non-stick frying pan or wok over a medium–high heat. Add the onion and peppers and stir-fry for 5 minutes. Add the garlic and curry paste and cook for 30 seconds more, stirring constantly.

Stir the coconut milk, lime leaves, nam pla and sugar into the pan and bring to a simmer. Cook for 2 minutes, stirring regularly. Add the cornflour liquid and then the fish pieces to the pan and reduce the heat slightly.

Cook the fish in the bubbling sauce for 4–5 minutes, gently shaking the pan, spooning over the sauce and turning the fish once until cooked through. Don't be too rough with the fish or it may break up. You will see it beginning to flake when it is ready.

Remove the pan from the heat and divide the curry between 2 warmed bowls. Scatter with fresh coriander if you like and serve with Broccoli and almond rice (page 279).

COOK'S TIPS

• I have started using blocks of coconut cream instead of coconut milk as it's difficult to find cans of coconut milk that don't contain stabilisers or other additives that could disrupt gut microbes. Coconut cream is pure coconut flesh that's been pressed into a block. It's available widely, in the world food section of the supermarket and in Asian stores. It's best to dissolve it in warm water before using, and I tend to add a little cornflour to make it taste more creamy. If you can't get hold of any, use half a well-mixed can of coconut milk instead.

• It's well worth searching out some fresh kaffir lime leaves as they make all the difference. (You can freeze the ones you don't use.) If using dry ones, add an extra couple to the sauce to help bring out the citrusy flavour.

MAKE A CHANGE

• Try making this curry with frozen prawns instead. Use cold-water prawns from the Atlantic rather than the plumper, deep pink warm-water prawns (tiger prawns) which are intensively farmed. Large cold-water prawns have lots more flavour and will defrost in less than an hour scattered over a plate at room temperature, or they can be thawed in the fridge overnight.

• If you really hate fish and there is nothing I can do to tempt you, make this dish with 1 very thinly sliced large, boneless, skinless chicken breast instead. Stir-fry with the curry paste and garlic until lightly coloured before adding the rest of the ingredients.

• It's easy to make this curry meat-free by stir frying 1 medium aubergine, cut into roughly 2.5cm chunks, in 1 tablespoon extra virgin olive oil for 2 minutes, or until lightly browned, before adding the remaining oil and the onion and peppers.

Pad Thai with prawns

Just as good as a takeaway pad Thai. Read the recipe carefully and get everything measured out and ready before you start as you need to be able to cook this dish quickly over a high heat. The slight caramelisation of the vegetables and noodles in the sweetly sour sauce is what gives it the deep savoury flavour.

SERVES 2 | **PREP:** 20 minutes | **COOK:** 6–8 minutes

85g soba noodles, wholewheat egg noodles or wide flat rice noodles
1 tbsp extra virgin olive oil, plus 1 tsp
1½ tbsp nam pla (Thai fish sauce) or dark soy sauce
juice of ½ lime (about 1 tbsp)
2 tsp light soft brown sugar or runny honey
1 small red onion, peeled, halved and cut into 8 wedges
1 small red or yellow pepper, deseeded and finely sliced
2 garlic cloves, peeled and finely chopped
1 large egg, well beaten
100g large cooked and peeled prawns (preferably cold-water and not farmed), thawed if frozen
25g roasted salted peanuts, roughly chopped
4 spring onions, trimmed and sliced
¼–½ tsp dried chilli flakes, depending on taste
20g bunch fresh coriander, leaves roughly chopped
lime wedges, for squeezing

Half-fill a large saucepan with water and bring to the boil. Add the noodles, return to the boil and cook for 2–3 minutes or until just tender, stirring occasionally. You may need to use a fork to stir and separate the noodles as they cook.

Drain the noodles in a colander and toss with the 1 teaspoon of oil to stop the strands sticking together, then put to one side. Mix the fish sauce or soy sauce, lime juice and sugar in a small bowl.

Pour the remaining tablespoon of oil into a large wok or non-stick frying pan and stir-fry the red onion and pepper over a medium heat for 2–3 minutes, or until softened and beginning to brown. Add the garlic and cook for a few seconds more. Push all the vegetables to one side of the pan.

Pour the beaten eggs into the pan and allow to cook into a thin omelette on the bottom. This should take 30–40 seconds. Just before the egg is completely set, use a wooden spoon to roughly chop it.

Immediately add the prawns, cooked noodles, peanuts, spring onions and fish sauce mixture. Increase the heat to its highest setting and stir-fry together for 2 minutes. Toss all the ingredients with tongs or two wooden spoons as you stir-fry to make sure everything is thoroughly hot and well mixed.

Add the chilli flakes and coriander and stir-fry for 2–3 minutes more until the noodles and eggs are lightly browned in places. Divide the pad Thai between warmed plates or bowls using tongs. Serve with extra fish sauce and soy sauce for seasoning.

MAKE A CHANGE

• For a vegetarian alternative, fry either 150g button mushrooms, cut in half, or well-drained tofu in a little oil until golden brown, then transfer to a plate until the noodles and spring onions are hot (omit the fish sauce). Return to the pan with the beansprouts and heat through.

• You can use roughly chopped cashew nuts or mixed nuts for this dish instead of the peanuts if you prefer. If you do end up opening a bag of nuts especially, store the ones you don't use immediately in a jar with a tight-fitting lid.

Meat-free meals

It should be no surprise to see so many meat-free dishes in this book, as large meat consumption has been linked to cancer and heart disease. That doesn't mean you have to cut it out altogether but switching to more plant-based foods will keep your fibre levels up and your gut microbes thriving. And, more importantly, by encouraging plenty of beneficial bacteria to flourish, you will help to crowd out the harmful microbes associated with illness, disease and weight gain.

By eating a meat-free supper at least three times a week during the plan, you will be able to build a repertoire of vegetarian dishes that you can return to again and again after the four weeks is up. If there is something that crops up on the plan that doesn't appeal, simply swap it for another dish that does – they're all designed to help feed your internal garden.

The selection of recipes here doesn't contain anything too scary in terms of unusual ingredients, but you will find you are eating plenty more foods that are high in fibre, particularly the prebiotic fermentable fibre, than you might have done in the past. If you are not used to eating this way, you might experience some bloating and wind to begin with as your body, and your microbes, adjust. If you find you are experiencing discomfort, simply cut down on the dried pulses, such as beans and lentils, and stick with more vegetable and rice-based dishes until things have settled. Remember to drink plenty of water as extra fibre can dehydrate you.

The recipes

One-pan pasta with broccoli and tomatoes

Veggie bolognese

Shepherdess pie

Veg-packed peppers

Smoky bean chilli

Beany nut burgers

Chickpea masala

Mixed vegetable and lentil curry

Sweet potato and spinach dhal

Green vegetable and barley risotto

Mediterranean vegetable lasagne

One-pan pasta with broccoli and tomatoes

A really easy supper for two, this colourful pasta dish is filling and very delicious. Add chilli to suit your own taste – I always plump for half a teaspoon but you may prefer to tread a bit more carefully first time round.

SERVES 2 | **PREP:** 5 minutes | **COOK:** 12 minutes

100g wholewheat dried spaghetti

150g broccoli, cut into small florets and halved, or asparagus, trimmed and cut into short lengths

150g cherry tomatoes, halved

2 garlic cloves, peeled and very thinly sliced

2 tbsp extra virgin olive oil

¼–½ tsp dried chilli flakes (depending on taste)

2 tbsp fresh lemon juice

sea salt and black pepper

25g Parmesan, finely grated

25g pine nuts

handful fresh basil leaves, roughly torn or shredded

Pour 500ml of water into a large wide-based sauté pan, deep frying pan or shallow casserole and bring to the boil.

Add the spaghetti to the boiling water, return to the boil and cook for 8 minutes, stirring occasionally. Add the broccoli, or asparagus, to the same pan and cook for 2 minutes more. By this time almost all of the water should have evaporated.

Add the tomatoes, garlic, olive oil, chilli flakes and lemon juice. Season with salt and pepper. Cook for 2–3 minutes, tossing with two wooden spoons until the spaghetti is lightly coated with the spices from the pan and the tomatoes are softened but still holding their shape.

Sprinkle over the Parmesan, scatter with pine nuts and basil leaves and toss together. Divide between the 2 warmed plates using tongs or a couple of forks. Drizzle with extra olive oil and sprinkle with more Parmesan to serve if you like. This tastes good with a punchy vinaigrette-dressed salad.

MAKE A CHANGE

• Any long pasta shape, such as tagliatelle or linguine, will work just as well as the spaghetti. And even short pasta shapes can be substituted – simply adjust the cooking times accordingly.

• If you like, you could add a can of drained tuna to the pasta. Simply flake the tuna into the pan once the tomatoes are cooked and heat with the pasta for 1 minute more, tossing very gently so it doesn't break up too much.

• Use extra vegetables too if you like, or stir in some sliced mushrooms along with the tomatoes.

Veggie bolognese

This delicious, fibre-rich bolognese is so good you won't miss the mince. It takes a little longer to prepare than a traditional recipe as you'll need to gather a few extra vegetables, but it's very easy and makes six generous servings, so you'll have a few handy in the freezer for another day. It also makes a brilliant base for veggie cottage pies and lasagne. I recommend using the red wine as it helps make the bolognese taste particularly rich and delicious.

SERVES 6 | **PREP:** 15 minutes | **COOK:** 50–55 minutes

100g dried puy or green lentils
100g dried split red lentils
2 tbsp extra virgin olive oil
1 medium red onion, peeled and finely chopped
2 garlic cloves, peeled and crushed
2 celery sticks, trimmed and finely sliced
2 medium carrots (about 200g), coarsely grated
1 medium courgette (about 150g), cut into roughly 1.5cm cubes
1 red or green pepper, deseeded and cut into roughly 1.5cm chunks

1 slender leek, trimmed and cut into roughly 5mm slices
250g chestnut mushrooms, sliced
400g can chopped tomatoes
750ml cold water
200ml red wine or extra water
4 tbsp tomato purée
2 tsp dried oregano or dried mixed herbs
1 vegetable stock cube
2 bay leaves, ideally fresh
sea salt and black pepper
grated Parmesan, to serve

Put the lentils in a bowl and cover with cold water; leave to stand. Heat the oil in a large, wide-based non-stick saucepan, flameproof casserole or deep sauté pan and gently fry the onion, garlic, celery, carrots, courgette and pepper for 10 minutes until softened, stirring regularly.

Drain the lentils in a sieve and stir into the vegetables. Add the leek, mushrooms, tomatoes, water, wine if using, tomato purée, oregano or mixed herbs, stock cube and bay leaves. Season with salt and pepper and bring to a gentle simmer.

Cover loosely with a lid and cook for 30 minutes, stirring

occasionally. Remove the lid and simmer for a further 10–15 minutes, or until the red lentils have completely softened and the sauce is thick. The puy lentils will retain much of their texture. Stir occasionally at the beginning and more regularly towards the end of the cooking time so it doesn't stick. And add a little extra water if the lentils soak up the first batch before they are quite tender. Adjust the seasoning to taste, making sure you are generous with the black pepper.

Serve with spaghetti, topped with freshly grated Parmesan cheese. A large mixed salad dressed with my Olive oil vinaigrette (page 292) goes very well and adds lots of useful antioxidants.

FREEZING TIP
Flat-freeze the cooked and cooled sauce in zip-seal bags for up to four months. Reheat from frozen in a wide-based non-stick saucepan, or microwave, with an extra splash of water, stirring regularly until piping hot throughout.

MAKE A CHANGE
• If you are a bit unsure whether you are ready for a full-on veggie bolognese, cut out the puy (green) lentils and brown 200–250g lean minced beef or lamb in the pan with the vegetables, adding a beef or lamb stock cube. That way, you'll have a fibre-rich bolognese that should be a bit gentler on your digestion.
• Use a pouch of cooked puy lentils or canned lentils if you can't find the dry kind in your local store and decrease the water by about 100ml.

FOLLOWING THE 28-DAY PLAN?

Make sure you freeze four portions of the bolognese for later in the plan. Flat-freeze in two zip-seal bags.

Shepherdess pie

A traditional recipe given a meat-free twist. Use two portions of the veggie bolognese and top with home-made mash potatoes with added leeks and cheese.

SERVES 2 | **PREP:** 10 minutes | **COOK:** 20–25 minutes

300g potatoes, ideally Maris Piper, peeled and cut into roughly 3cm chunks
1 slender leek, trimmed and thinly sliced
1 tbsp extra virgin olive oil

50ml semi-skimmed or whole milk
25g butter
25g Cheddar, or any other hard cheese, coarsely grated
2 portions frozen veggie bolognese, defrosted in the fridge overnight

Put the potatoes in a medium saucepan and cover with cold water. Bring the water to the boil, then reduce the heat slightly and cook the potatoes for 15–20 minutes, or until very tender. Preheat the oven to 220°C/fan oven 200°C/gas 7.

While the potatoes are cooking, heat the oil in a medium non-stick pan and fry the leek gently for 3–4 minutes or until softened. Drain the potatoes and mash with the milk and butter until smooth. Add the leeks, mix well and season to taste.

Put the veggie bolognese into a small ovenproof dish and top with the leek mash. Sprinkle with the cheese and bake for 20–25 minutes or until nicely browned and hot throughout.

MAKE A CHANGE
• Instead of white potatoes, try topping the pies with mashed celeriac, squash or sweet potatoes
• Cook 2–3 finely sliced Jerusalem artichokes with the potatoes for an extra prebiotic boost.

Veg-packed peppers

Use leftover portions of veggie bolognese to make these simple stuffed peppers. The serving is generous, making a hearty supper for 2 or a light lunch for 4 people. I always cook in the microwave because they are so handy taken to work, but the oven method works well too. Top with a drizzle of fresh basil pesto and serve with a large mixed salad if you like.

SERVES 2 | **PREP:** 5 minutes | **COOK:** 50-60 minutes

2 portions frozen veggie bolognese,
   defrosted in the fridge overnight
2 large peppers (any colour)
25g grated or cubed cheese
   (ideally unpasteurised/raw milk),
   grated, cubed or crumbled

Preheat the oven to 220°C/fan oven 200°C/gas 7. Cut the peppers in half from stalk to base and remove the seeds. Place the peppers in a small oiled roasting tin or ovenproof dish, cut side up.

Divide the bolognese mixture between the peppers, piling on top. Cover with a large piece of kitchen foil and bake for 50-60 minutes or until the peppers are tender and the filling is hot throughout.

Alternatively, put the stuffed peppers in a microwavable dish, cover and cook on HIGH for about 5 minutes.

Sprinkle the peppers with cheese just before serving.

Smoky bean chilli

A really hearty chilli that even committed meat-eaters will enjoy.
It's full of fibre-rich beans and colourful, antioxidant-packed
veggies. You can use any beans that you have handy or use up
any that are leftover from other meals. Serve with wholegrain
rice and raw vegetable salsas for an extra vitamin boost and
don't forget to top with probiotic live yogurt.

SERVES 4 | **PREP:** 15 minutes | **COOK:** 30–35 minutes

2 tbsp extra virgin olive oil

2 medium red onions, peeled and
thinly sliced

1 yellow or orange pepper,
deseeded and cut into roughly
2cm chunks

1 red pepper, deseeded and cut into
roughly 2cm chunks

1 medium sweet potato (about
300g), cut into roughly 3cm
chunks

2 tsp ground coriander

2 tsp ground cumin

2 tsp ground turmeric

2 garlic cloves, peeled and crushed

400g can chopped tomatoes

2 tbsp tomato purée

1–2 tbsp chipotle paste (from a jar),
depending on taste (see tip)

400g can mixed beans

400g can red kidney beans

500ml vegetable stock (made with
1 stock cube)

sea salt and black pepper

full-fat live natural yogurt and rice
to serve

Heat the oil in a large, deep, wide-based saucepan or flameproof
casserole. Add the onions to the pan and cook for 5 minutes,
stirring. Scatter the peppers and sweet potato into the pan.
Stir-fry with the onions for 3–5 minutes, or until beginning to
soften and lightly brown. Sprinkle over the ground coriander,
cumin, turmeric and garlic and cook for a few seconds more,
stirring constantly.

Add the chopped tomatoes, tomato purée, chipotle paste and
beans to the pan and stir in the stock. Season with a large pinch of
salt and lots of ground black pepper. Bring the liquid to a simmer
and cook for 25–30 minutes or until all the vegetables are tender,
stirring regularly. (Add an extra splash of water if necessary.)
Adjust the seasoning to taste.

Top the chilli with spoonfuls of live yogurt and serve with freshly cooked mixed rice, sliced avocado, or Zingy avocado salsa (page 269) and Fresh tomato salsa (page 268).

FREEZING TIP
Flat-freeze the cooked and cooled chilli in zip-seal bags for up to four months. Defrost in the fridge overnight. Reheat in a wide-based non-stick saucepan, or microwave, stirring regularly until piping hot throughout.

MAKE A CHANGE
• This delicious bean stew gets its smoky flavour from chipotle paste, made from smoked jalapeno peppers. You should find it in the Mexican or world food section of the supermarket, but if you can't find any in your local store, add 2 tsp smoked paprika (not hot smoked) and ½–1 tsp hot chilli powder at the same time as the other dried spices instead.
• If you are a bit unsure whether you are ready for a full-on veggie chilli, omit one can of beans and brown 200–250g lean minced beef or lamb in the pan with the vegetables before adding the spices and all the remaining ingredients, and use beef or lamb stock instead of vegetable stock. See how your gut responds and if all is good, make without the mince next time. Leftover mince can be wrapped tightly in a freezer bag and frozen for up to three months. Thaw overnight in the freezer and then use as you would fresh mince.
• If you like mushrooms, add 100g, halved or sliced, to the pan at the same time as the pepper and sweet potato.

FOLLOWING THE 28-DAY PLAN?

Make sure you freeze two portions of the chilli for later in the plan. Flat-freeze in one zip-seal bag.

Beany nut burgers

Bean burgers can be a tricky thing to make, but this Moroccan-inspired recipe works brilliantly. You will need a food processor to do the mixing for you but it doesn't take long. The burgers are also delicious served cold, so are brilliant for packed lunches. Or serve these burgers as a main meal with a large mixed salad and lots of probiotic live yogurt and mint dip.

SERVES 2 | **PREP:** 15 minutes | **COOK:** 8 minutes

1 small red onion, peeled and roughly chopped
1 large garlic clove, peeled and halved
25g mixed nuts (such as Brazils, almonds, hazelnuts, walnuts and pecan nuts)
2 tsp ground cumin
2 tsp ground coriander
freshly ground pepper
1 tsp flaked sea salt

400g can mixed beans, rinsed and drained
25g plain or wholemeal plain flour
20g bunch fresh coriander with stalks
1 tbsp fresh lemon juice
3 tbsp extra virgin olive oil

For the minted yogurt sauce:
100g full-fat live natural yogurt
10g bunch fresh mint, leaves finely chopped

To make the yogurt sauce, mix the yogurt and mint in a bowl, cover and chill until needed.

To make the burgers, put the onion, garlic, nuts, spices and salt into a food processor and add lots of freshly ground black pepper. Blitz until the mixture is as smooth as possible. Add the mixed beans, flour, coriander and lemon juice and blitz until the mixture comes together to make a thick paste. It shouldn't be too smooth as you are looking for some texture to give the burgers a bit of bite.

Form the mixture into 4 balls and flatten into burgers, just under 2cm deep. Heat 2 tablespoons of the oil in a medium non-stick frying pan over a low heat and cook the burgers on one side for 3–5 minutes, checking they are crispy and browned on the bottom but not burnt.

Add the remaining oil to the pan and turn the burgers over.

Cook on the other side for about 3 minutes or until nicely browned and hot throughout. (Keep the heat low, so they don't burn.) Serve with a large mixed salad and the minted yogurt sauce.

FREEZING TIP

Freeze the uncooked burgers on a baking tray lined with foil until solid then transfer to a freezer bag and freeze for up to one month. Thaw in the fridge overnight and cook as above.

COOK'S TIPS

• When blending the ingredients in a food processor, you may need to remove the lid and push the mixture down a couple of times with a rubber spatula until the right consistency is reached. (If you have a small food processor, you may need to blend the mixture in two batches.)
• I use canned beans to save time and it's best to choose mixed canned beans for variety, although you could use half a 400g tin of chickpeas and half a tin of 400g red kidney beans if you prefer. Rinse the beans in a sieve under cold running water and drain well before using. If using the beans for a more saucy recipe, you can omit the rinsing and draining step as the canning water contains extra nutrients.

MAKE A CHANGE

If you don't have a food processor, make some quick spiced beans instead. Simply heat the oil and fry the onion and garlic until softened. Add the spices and cook for a few seconds before stirring in the beans, coriander and lemon juice. Heat through on the hob for a few minutes then season to taste with salt and pepper and serve with salad.

Chickpea masala

This is one of my favourite veggie curries and is packed with flavour. The onions, garlic and chickpeas are full of fermentable soluble fibre. The sauce should be slightly sour but rich and warming. Serve with minted yogurt and a tomato and onion relish.

SERVES 2 | **PREP:** 15 minutes | **COOK:** 40 minutes

2 tbsp extra virgin olive oil

1 medium onion, peeled and finely sliced

2 garlic cloves, peeled and crushed

15g chunk fresh root ginger, peeled and finely grated

1 green chilli, finely chopped (deseeded first if you prefer)

1 tsp cumin seeds

1 tbsp medium curry powder

¼ tsp hot chilli powder

1 tsp ground turmeric

227g can chopped tomatoes

2 tbsp tomato purée

½ tsp flaked sea salt

400g can chickpeas

300ml cold water

1 tbsp fresh lemon juice

bunch coriander, chopped, plus extra leaves to garnish

Heat the oil in a large wide-based saucepan. Add the onion and fry gently for 5 minutes, or until softened and lightly browned, stirring occasionally.

Stir in the garlic, ginger, chilli and cumin seeds and fry together for 2 minutes, stirring constantly. Sprinkle over the curry powder, hot chilli powder and turmeric and continue to stir over a low heat for 2 minutes without burning. If the spices begin to stick, add a splash of cold water and continue cooking.

Tip the tomatoes into the pan and stir in the tomato purée and salt. Bring to the boil and cook for 4–5 minutes, stirring constantly until the sauce is very thick. This will help intensify the flavours.

Add the chickpeas and water. Reduce the heat, so the sauce simmers gently. Cover loosely and cook for 25 minutes, stirring regularly until the chickpeas are very tender, the sauce is thick and the spices have mellowed. If the sauce becomes too thick before the time is up, add a little more water.

Season and add the lemon juice to taste. Continue to cook for 2 minutes more. Stir in the coriander and serve with Minted yogurt with cucumber (page 270) and Fresh tomato salsa (page 268).

FREEZING TIP

Freeze the cooled curry in zip-seal bags or foil containers for up to three months. Cook from frozen or thaw in the fridge overnight. Reheat thoroughly in a large saucepan, stirring regularly until piping hot.

Mixed vegetable and lentil curry

This is a vegetarian dish that even committed meat lovers will enjoy. It's packed with vegetables and very easy to make. The onions, garlic and peas are all high in prebiotic fibre, so it makes for especially gut-happy microbes when served symbiotically with probiotic yogurt. Paneer is an Indian cheese that cooks beautifully and retains its texture, but you could use stir-fried chicken breast or prawns instead.

SERVES 4 | **PREP:** 20 minutes | **COOK:** 35–40 minutes

300g potatoes, ideally Maris Piper, peeled and cut into roughly 2cm chunks

½ cauliflower (around 300g), cut into small florets and halved

2 medium carrots, peeled and cut into roughly 5mm diagonal slices or batons

250g small chestnut mushrooms, halved, or quartered if large

2 tbsp extra virgin olive oil

40g butter

2 large onions, (around 350g/12oz), peeled and coarsely grated or very finely chopped

15g chunk fresh root ginger, peeled and finely grated

3 garlic cloves, peeled and crushed

2 tbsp medium curry powder

227g can chopped tomatoes

50g dried red split lentils

2 tbsp mango chutney

500ml vegetable or chicken stock (made with 1 cube)

100g frozen peas or young spinach, or a mixture of both

full-fat live natural yogurt, to serve

A third fill a large saucepan with cold water and add the potatoes. Bring to the boil. Add cauliflower and carrots, and cook for 3 minutes. Drain in a colander and set aside.

Heat 1 tbsp of the oil a large non-stick sautee pan, wide-based saucepan or flame-proof casserole. Fry the mushrooms over a medium-high heat for 3-4 minutes, or until golden brown, turning occasionally and adding a little more oil if necessary. Tip onto a plate and return the pan to the heat.

Add the remaining oil and butter and the onions and cook over a medium heat for 10 minutes or until the onions are well softened and lightly browned, stirring regularly. Stir in the ginger and garlic and curry powder cook for a minute more, stirring constantly.

Add the tomatoes, lentils, mango chutney and stock to the spiced onions and bring to a gentle simmer. Cook for 15 minutes or until the lentils are very soft, stirring occasionally.

When the curry sauce is ready, return the mushrooms to the pan with the onions, add the part-cooked vegetables and simmer gently for 5 minutes more, stirring occasionally. If the sauce thickens too much, add a splash of water.

Stir in the peas or spinach and cook for 2–3 minutes more. Serve topped with full-fat live natural yogurt. You can add small portions of cooked wholegrain rice but it shouldn't be necessary as the curry already contains potatoes.

FREEZING TIP
Flat-freeze the cooked and cooled curry in zip-seal bags for up to two months. Cook from frozen or thaw in the fridge overnight. Reheat in a microwave or large wide-based saucepan, stirring gently until piping hot throughout.

MAKE A CHANGE
• Instead of mushrooms, try using 225g Paneer or 2 x 150g boneless chicken breast, cut into 2.5cm cubes. Paneer is an Indian cheese that cooks beautifully and retains its texture. Add to the curry sauce at the same time as the part-cooked vegetables.
• Use 1 tsp caster sugar instead of the mango chutney, or leave it out, if you prefer.
• This curry is quite mild, so if you prefer a spicier curry, add a finely chopped green or red chilli, or ½ tsp dried chilli flakes, after the mango chutney.
• If you don't have medium curry powder handy, use 2 tsp ground cumin, 2 tsp ground coriander, 1 tsp ground turmeric and ¼ tsp hot chilli powder instead.

FOLLOWING THE 28-DAY PLAN?

Make sure you freeze two portions of this curry for later in the plan. Flat-freeze in one zip-seal bag.

Sweet potato and spinach dhal

This lightly curried dhal makes a brilliant lunch or light supper, served with natural yogurt and wholemeal flatbreads (page 296). Packed in a suitable container, it can be warmed up at work, too. Alternatively, serve it alongside another curry to make the meal go further. I use curry powder for this recipe but you could use a medium curry paste instead.

SERVES 4 | **PREP:** 15 minutes | **COOK:** 30–35 minutes

2 tbsp extra virgin olive oil
2 medium onions, peeled and thinly sliced
2 garlic cloves, peeled and crushed
20g chunk fresh root ginger, peeled and finely grated
2 tbsp medium curry powder
200g dried red split lentils
500g sweet potatoes (about 1–2 large), cut into roughly 3cm chunks

1 tsp flaked sea salt, plus extra to season
1 litre water
1 long green or red chilli, thinly sliced (optional)
1–2 tbsp fresh lime or lemon juice, to taste
black pepper
full-fat live natural yogurt and lime or lemon wedges, to serve

Heat the oil in a large non-stick saucepan and fry the onion over a medium heat for 5 minutes, or until softened and very lightly browned, stirring frequently. Stir in the garlic, ginger and curry powder and cook for 1 minute more.

Add the lentils, sweet potatoes, salt, water and sliced chilli, if using. Bring the water to the boil and spoon off and discard any froth that rises to the surface of the pan. Reduce the heat, cover the pan loosely with a lid and cook for about 25 minutes, or until the lentils and sweet potato are tender, stirring occasionally. Add an extra splash of water if the dhal thickens too much before the lentils are ready.

Stir in the lime or lemon juice and adjust the salt and pepper to taste. Serve with lots of full-fat live natural yogurt or my Minted yogurt and cucumber (page 270) and Fresh tomato salsa (page 268).

FREEZING TIP
Flat-freeze the cooked and cooled curry in zip-seal bags for up to two months. Cook from frozen or thaw in the fridge overnight. Reheat in a large wide-based saucepan, stirring gently until piping hot throughout.

MAKE A CHANGE
If you don't have any curry powder to hand, use 2 tsp ground cumin, 2 tsp ground coriander, ½ tsp hot chilli powder, 1 tsp ground turmeric and ½ tsp ground black pepper. Or, grind the whole spices in a pestle and mortar instead.

Green vegetable and barley risotto

Pearl barley makes a lovely alternative risotto that manages to be both filling and light – far less stodgy than a traditionally made risotto and I think far more delicious too. Barley is full of soluble fibre that gut microbes love and has been linked to good heart health.

SERVES 2 | **PREP:** 25 minutes | **COOK:** 35 minutes

1 tbsp extra virgin olive oil
1 medium onion, peeled and very finely chopped
1 medium leek, trimmed and finely sliced
2 garlic cloves, peeled and crushed
100g pearl barley
75ml white wine, vermouth or extra chicken stock

1 vegetable or chicken stock cube
800ml water
100g fine asparagus spears, trimmed and halved
50g frozen peas
40g Parmesan, finely grated
sea salt and black pepper

Heat the oil in large non-stick saucepan and gently fry the onion for 3 minutes, stirring occasionally. Add the leek and cook for 2 minutes more, stirring. Next, add the garlic and cook for a few seconds, stirring constantly.

Stir in the pearl barley and then add the wine or vermouth, if using, and let bubble for a few seconds before adding the stock cube and water.

Bring to the boil, stirring occasionally, then reduce the heat slightly, cover with a lid and simmer for 25 minutes, or until tender. Stir occasionally, especially towards the end of the cooking time. Take some of the barley out of the pan and check that it's soft. If not, add an extra splash of water and cook for a few minutes more.

Stir in the asparagus and peas and cook for a further 5 minutes or until the green vegetables are just cooked, stirring constantly. Remove the pan from the heat and stir in half the Parmesan. Season with salt and pepper to taste. Spoon into bowls and top with more grated Parmesan just before serving. A lightly dressed mixed leaf salad is a delicious accompaniment to this dish.

MAKE A CHANGE
You can add leftover shredded cooked chicken to the risotto at the same time as the asparagus and peas if you like. It's a great way of using up chicken from a Sunday roast. Try topping with cubed or crumbled unpasteurised (raw milk) cheese too.

Mediterranean vegetable lasagne

This delicious lasagne is made with chunky vegetables in a rich, garlicky tomato sauce. It does take a while to prepare but the recipe makes enough for six servings and freezes brilliantly. Serve with a large mixed salad.

SERVES 6 | **PREP:** 25 minutes | **COOK:** 50–60 minutes

1 small aubergine (about 250g), cut into roughly 2.5cm chunks

2 medium courgettes (about 400g total weight), quartered lengthways and cut into roughly 2cm chunks

2 yellow or red peppers, deseeded and cut into roughly 2cm chunks

1 medium red onion, peeled and cut into thin wedges

3 tbsp extra virgin olive oil

sea salt and black pepper

4 garlic cloves, peeled and finely sliced

400g can chopped tomatoes

75g dried red split lentils

3 tbsp tomato purée

2 tsp dried oregano

1 fresh bay leaf or 2 dried bay leaves

150ml red wine or extra water

1 vegetable stock cube

2 tsp sugar, any kind (optional)

300ml cold water

6 dried lasagne sheets, ideally wholewheat

For the cheese sauce:

50g butter

50g plain flour

600ml semi-skimmed or whole milk

50g Parmesan cheese, finely grated

100g young spinach leaves

Put the aubergine, courgettes, peppers and onion in a large bowl. Pour over the oil and season with salt and lots of ground black pepper. Toss well together.

Place a large non-stick frying pan or wok over a high heat and stir-fry the vegetables in 3 batches for 1–2 minutes, or until nicely browned, putting the first 2 batches in a large saucepan or flame-proof casserole while the third batch is cooked. Pre-browning the vegetables like this will add lots of flavour to the lasagne.

Add the garlic to the final batch of vegetables and cook for a few seconds more before adding to the rest of the vegetables.

Add the tomatoes, lentils, tomato purée, oregano, bay leaf, red wine, crumbled stock cube, sugar and water. Bring the liquid to a simmer, then reduce the heat and cook for 15 minutes, or until the vegetables are softened and the sauce is thick, stirring occasionally. Season with salt and pepper. Preheat the oven to 200°C/fan oven 180°C/gas 6.

While the vegetables are cooking, make the cheese sauce. Put the butter, flour and milk in a medium saucepan and whisk over a low–medium heat for 4–5 minutes or until the sauce is smooth and thickened. (Use a silicone-covered whisk if using a non-stick pan to prevent scratches.) Using a wooden spoon, stir in half the Parmesan cheese and the spinach leaves, one handful at a time, and season with salt and pepper to taste.

Spread half the vegetables over the base of a 2.5-litre shallow ovenproof lasagne dish (or 2–3 smaller dishes), cover with dried lasagne sheets. Repeat the layers, ending in the pasta. Pour over the cheese sauce and sprinkle with the remaining Parmesan. Bake for 25–30 minutes or until golden brown and hot throughout. Stand for 5–10 minutes before cutting. Serve with a large mixed salad and olive oil vinaigrette.

FREEZING TIP

Freeze the cooked and cooled lasagne in one or two shallow freezer-proof and ovenproof containers (foil containers are good here). It will keep in the freezer for up to three months. Thaw overnight in the fridge. Reheat in a preheated oven at 200°C/fan oven 180°C/gas 6, covered loosely with foil, for 20–30 minutes or until hot throughout. Alternatively, microwave individual portions on covered plates for 4–5 minutes, or until hot.

FOLLOWING THE 28-DAY PLAN?

Cut the cooked lasagne into 6 portions. Serve 2 as your evening meal and put the other 4 in individual freezer-proof dishes. Cover and freeze for later in the plan.

Breakfasts and brunches

Despite what you might have read in recent years, there is absolutely no need to eat breakfast unless you want to. In fact, giving your digestion a nice long break between meals is actually very good for it. Breakfast is meant to be literally 'breaking the fast', and leaving twelve hours or ideally longer between your last meal and the next helps your stomach and small intestine to completely empty. Depending on your genes, you may fancy breakfast first thing or be happier to wait and eat a bit later. Whichever it is, listen to your body and eat when you are hungry rather than adhering to outdated information.

For the 28-day plan, I've made breakfast suggestions for you, but do feel free to swap them around to fit in with your lifestyle. I've suggested oat, fruit and yogurt-based breakfasts on four days of the week, as they all contain a good mix of prebiotic fermentable fibre, polyphenol-filled fruit and nuts and probiotic yogurt, making them the ideal gut-happy choice. And don't forget about including kefir too if you can (see page 46). This type of breakfast is also easy to transport if you work away from home and don't fancy eating before you leave. There are a couple of egg-based breakfasts included each week too – something simple midweek and a more involved brunch recipe for the weekend. Swap them around to suit yourself.

The recipes

Yogurt and fruit with oat and nut crunch

Oat and nut crunch

Hot or cold oats

Overnight muesli with berries

Boiled eggs with asparagus soldiers

Poached eggs with smashed avocado

Scrambled eggs with asparagus

Mediterranean brunch eggs

Leek and cheese omelette

Apple pancakes with blueberries and banana

Lower-sugar plum freezer jam

Yogurt cheese

DID YOU KNOW?
A special bacterium has been identified that has been shown
to clean up the gut lining and have an impact on weight loss. If
weight loss is your goal, I suggest you rest your gut for at least
twelve hours overnight and cut out snacks. It's also a good idea
to occasionally have a gentle fast, by sticking to just a couple of
smaller meals one day a week, to give your microbes a chance to
do their job properly.

BACON AND SAUSAGES
While you are following the 28-day plan, you won't see any
processed meat products, such as bacon and sausages, but you
can reintroduce them after the time is up. It's best to indulge
only occasionally, though – no more than once a week if possible
– as frequent consumption of processed meats is connected to
increased risks of cancer and heart disease.

Yogurt and fruit with oat and nut crunch

There are different ways to enjoy the easiest combination of ingredients for a gut-happy breakfast. A few spoonfuls of full-fat live yogurt, topped with a handful of fresh berries, some wholegrain porridge oats, a few chopped nuts and a sprinkling of seeds is the simplest way, but you can also try this recipe, containing all the right ingredients.

SERVES 2 | **PREP:** 5 minutes

200g full-fat live natural yogurt
200g mixed fruit, either fresh,
   frozen and thawed or poached
50g oat and nut crunch (page 235)

Divide the yogurt between two bowls and top with the fruit. Sprinkle over the oat and nut crunch and serve.

MAKE A CHANGE
You can take this breakfast to work with you by layering into small, sturdy jars. Start with the yogurt, top with the fruit and end with the oat and nut crunch. Keep cool.

FOLLOWING THE 28-DAY PLAN?

Buy fruit that you can eat over 2–3 days on the plan. Fresh berries are particularly good as they contain a range of antioxidants. Frozen berries are a less-expensive alternative too. And don't forget stewed fruits that can be poached in a saucepan or the microwave until softened. Try to use naturally sweet fruit, so you aren't tempted to add sugar.

Oat and nut crunch

This crunchy, oaty topping is very easy to make and can be stored in an airtight jar for up to two weeks. Sprinkle onto yogurt and berries for breakfast or use as a topping for stewed fruit.

SERVES 8 | **PREP:** 5 minutes | **COOK:** 15 minutes

30g runny honey (about 2 tbsp)
2 tbsp extra virgin olive oil
1 tsp ground cinnamon
100g jumbo oats

50g mixed nuts, such as almonds, hazelnuts and Brazil nuts, roughly chopped
25g mixed seeds, such as pumpkin, sunflower and sesame

Preheat the oven to 170°C/fan oven 150°C/gas 3. Heat the honey and oil together in a medium saucepan until warm and runny. Take off the hob and stir in the cinnamon and oats until thoroughly mixed. Scatter evenly over a large baking tray and bake for 10 minutes.

Carefully take the tray out of the oven and stir in the nuts. Return to the oven for a further 10 minutes or until golden brown. Leave to cool and crisp up on the tray. Stir in the seeds. Store in an airtight jar for up to two weeks.

Hot or cold oats

Oats make a filling breakfast and are full of gut-healthy soluble fibre. Sometimes I don't feel like a bowl of hot porridge but oats cold as a simple muesli is great. It also means I can take breakfast with me if I'm working away from home.

SERVES 2 | **PREP:** 5 minutes | **COOK:** 4 minutes

25g mixed nuts
10g raisins or other dried fruit
1 just-ripe medium banana, sliced
65g jumbo porridge oats
250ml semi-skimmed or whole milk
150ml water (if needed)
2 tsp mixed seeds, such as pumpkin, sunflower, sesame and linseed

150g fresh or frozen mixed berries, such as strawberries, raspberries and blueberries, thawed if frozen (optional)
2-4 tbsp full-fat live natural yogurt (optional)

Roughly chop any of the larger nuts in your selection - probably the pecan nuts and Brazils, if using.

If serving the oats hot, place in a non-stick saucepan with the nuts, raisins, banana, milk and water and cook over a low–medium heat for about 5 minutes, stirring constantly until rich and creamy. Divide between two bowls and serve topped with mixed seeds, berries and yogurt if you like.

If serving cold, mix the nuts and raisins with the oats and divide between two bowls. Pour over 200ml of milk (you won't need it all). Top with the sliced banana and seeds, mixed berries if using, and the yogurt.

MAKE A CHANGE
Look out for packs of mixed rolled and flaked wholegrains, combined to make home made mueslis and porridge. They'll be in the wholefood or breakfast section of the supermarket and can be swapped for any of the plain porridge oats used here, adding even more diversity and plenty for your gut microbes to feast on. You'll find you'll need about half the liquid called for in the recipe if using a combination of grains.

Overnight muesli with berries

Sometimes called Bircher muesli, soaking oats overnight makes them particularly luscious and mixing with grated apple, berries, nuts and yogurt will give your gut microbes a useful cocktail of polyphenols, fermentable soluble fibre and plenty of probiotic bacteria. Even if you don't have time to soak the oats overnight, just 30 minutes or so will be enough to soften them considerably. I like to add the frozen berries to my muesli, but you can keep them for spooning on top if you like, or swap for fresh.

SERVES 2 | **PREP:** 10 minutes, plus several hours chilling

150g frozen mixed berries
1 eating apple, well washed
50g jumbo porridge oats
20g mixed seeds, such as sunflower, pumpkin, linseed and sesame
25g mixed nuts, such as Brazils, hazelnuts, almonds, pecans and walnuts, roughly chopped if large
1 tbsp runny honey
100g full-fat live natural yogurt
100ml semi-skimmed or whole milk

Put the berries in a bowl and thaw for 2–3 hours, or overnight in the fridge. (You can also thaw in the microwave on the defrost setting for about 5 minutes but do not allow to heat.)
Coarsely grate the apple without peeling, avoiding the core. Put into a bowl and add the oats, seeds, nuts, honey, yogurt, milk and half the berries. Mix well together. Cover and chill for several hours or overnight.

Spoon the muesli into two bowls or sturdy containers if taking to work and top with the remaining berries.

Boiled eggs with smoked salmon and asparagus soldiers

Boiled eggs make a great breakfast and useful snack. These ones are served with freshly cooked prebiotic asparagus spears instead of a slice of buttered toast for dipping and can be eaten hot or cold. Serve with slices of smoked salmon if you like; ideally organic.

SERVES 2 | **PREP:** 3 minutes | **COOK:** 7 minutes

2 large fridge-cold eggs
200g asparagus spears
4 smoked salmon slices (about 75g)
lemon wedges, for squeezing

Half-fill a small saucepan with water and bring to the boil. Gently add the eggs to the water and return to the boil. (If the eggs are added too quickly, the shells could crack.) Cook the eggs for 7 minutes for a soft-boiled egg.

While the eggs are cooking, half-fill a small frying pan with water and bring to a simmer. Trim the ends off the asparagus, add to the water and return to the boil. Cook the spears for 2–5 minutes or until just tender. Lift out with tongs and divide between two plates, adding a slice of smoked salmon and a lemon wedge.

Put the eggs in egg cups and place on the same plates. Cut off the tops. Serve with the smoked salmon and warm asparagus for dipping. Squeeze a little lemon juice over the salmon if you like.

Poached eggs with smashed avocado

This colourful breakfast packs a nutritious punch and is hugely popular. I like to serve mine with balsamic tomatoes too.

SERVES 2 | **PREP:** 10 minutes | **COOK:** 10 minutes

1 small, ripe avocado
½ long red chilli, finely chopped, or
   ¼ tsp dried chilli flakes
1 tsp fresh lime juice
sea salt and black pepper
2 large very fresh, fridge-cold eggs

2 slices sourdough or wholegrain
   bread
2 tsp mixed seeds, such as
   sunflower, pumpkin, linseed and
   sesame seeds
1 tsp extra virgin olive oil

Cut the avocado in half and remove the stone. Slide a large metal spoon around each half of the avocado to scoop out the flesh. Put the avocado in a bowl and, using a fork, mash with the chilli and lime juice. Season to taste.

Pour 5cm of cold water into a medium saucepan and bring to a very gentle simmer. Stir the water with a wooden spoon. Break the eggs into the pan, one at a time. Cook for 2½–3 minutes or until the whites are set and the yolks remain runny. While the eggs are cooking, toast the bread and spread with the avocado mash.

Drain the eggs with a slotted spoon and place on top of the toast. Sprinkle with the seeds and drizzle with the oil. Serve immediately.

MAKE A CHANGE
When you have a bit more time, serve these eggs with my Balsamic tomatoes. Simply gently fry 150g halved cherry tomatoes in 2 tsp of extra virgin olive oil for 2-3 minutes over a medium heat until softened, stirring regularly. Remove from the heat, add with 1 teaspoon of good balsamic vinegar, and season with a little salt and lots of freshly ground black pepper.

Scrambled eggs with asparagus

A luxurious breakfast for a lazy weekend. Serving asparagus alongside the eggs brings a good dose of prebiotic fibre to the dish. You can add smoked salmon or wafer-thin slices of Parma ham if you like.

SERVES 2 | **PREP:** 5 minutes | **COOK:** 2-3 minutes

4 large, fridge-cold eggs
15g butter
1 tsp extra virgin olive oil
100g asparagus, trimmed into roughly 3cm lengths
1 spring onion, trimmed and finely sliced

2 slices wholegrain or sourdough bread
4 smoked salmon slices (about 75g) or 4 slices Parma Ham (optional)
sea salt and black pepper

Beat the eggs in a bowl using a whisk until well combined. Season with a pinch of salt and lots of black pepper.

Melt the butter with the oil in a medium non-stick saucepan over a low heat. Add the asparagus and cook for 3-4 minutes or until just tender, stirring regularly. Add the spring onion and cook for a few seconds more, stirring constantly.

Pour the beaten eggs into the pan and cook very gently for 1½-2 minutes, stirring regularly until the eggs are softly scrambled. Remove from the heat.

While the eggs are cooking, toast the bread and cut in half. Divide between two warmed plates. Spoon the scrambled eggs over the toast, add slices of smoked salmon or Parma ham, if you like and season with a little more black pepper.

Mediterranean brunch eggs

A fantastically delicious one-pan dish that can be served straight from the pan at the table – perfect for a leisurely weekend breakfast or brunch. It's very easy to increase the number of servings to four by using whole cans of tomatoes and beans and adding extra eggs and cheese. If you don't have any feta handy, either leave out all together or swap for another cheese and coarsely grate on top.

SERVES 2 | **PREP:** 10 minutes | **COOK:** 20 minutes

2 tbsp extra virgin olive oil
1 medium red onion, peeled and
   thinly sliced
1 yellow pepper, deseeded and
   thinly sliced
1 medium courgette, cut into
   roughly 1.5cm chunks
2 garlic cloves, peeled and crushed
1 tsp hot smoked paprika
227g can chopped tomatoes
120g canned red kidney beans (half
   a 400g can)

1 tsp dried mixed herbs or dried
   oregano
15g bunch fresh coriander, leaves
   roughly chopped, plus extra to
   garnish
2 very fresh, large fridge-cold eggs
50g feta cheese or any
   unpasteurised (raw milk) cheese,
   such as goat's cheese, crumbled
   or coarsely grated (optional)
sea salt and black pepper
full-fat live Greek yogurt, to serve

Heat the oil in a medium non-stick frying pan. Add the onion, pepper and courgette and fry gently for 8-10 minutes or until lightly browned, stirring regularly. Add the garlic and paprika and cook for a few seconds more, stirring constantly.

Add the tomatoes, beans and dried herbs to the pan. Season with a little salt and lots of ground black pepper. Cook over a medium heat for 3–4 minutes, or until fairly thick, stirring regularly. Stir in the coriander and season with salt and lots of ground black pepper.

Make two holes in the tomato and bean mixture with a wooden spoon, and break an egg into each one. Season with black pepper, sprinkle with feta if using, cover with a lid or large piece of foil and cook for 3–5 minutes, or until the white has set and the yolk is hot but runny. Garnish with more coriander and serve topped with spoonfuls of yogurt.

COOK'S TIP
• Make sure your yogurt is made with lots of lovely live cultures (bacteria) – simply check on the label.
• The leftover beans can be stored in a covered bowl in the fridge and used for salads, stews and curries, or frozen tightly wrapped. If you need to use a 400g can of chopped tomatoes, transfer to a small bowl and keep covered in the fridge for up to three days or freeze what's leftover in a small freezer bag and add to Italian-style sauces and stews.

Leek and cheese omelette

This simple omelette makes a lovely weekend breakfast or lunch for one. The leek brings lots of prebiotic fermentable fibre and the unpasteurised cheese adds a boost of live bacteria. It's a great way of using up small pieces of cheese, so add any that need to be finished.

SERVES 1 | **PREP:** 5 minutes | **COOK:** 5 minutes

1 tsp extra virgin olive oil
10g butter
1 slender leek, trimmed and cut into 5mm slices
2 large eggs, beaten
6 cherry tomatoes, cut in half
20g unpasteurised (raw milk) cheese, such as goat's cheese; Roquefort, Combé, Gruyère; rind removed
sea salt and black pepper
mixed salad with olive oil vinaigrette, to serve

Melt the butter with the oil in a medium non-stick pan (it should have a diameter of no more than 18–20cm measured across the bottom or your omelette will be very flat) and gently fry the leek for 3–4 minutes, turning every now and then until just softened.

Beat the eggs and season with ground black pepper. Pour the eggs over the leek and allow to run around the pan. Using a wooden spoon, draw the cooked egg in from the edges towards the centre of the pan 5–6 times, working your way around the pan and letting the raw egg flow into the space that it leaves. This will help the egg become thicker and 'fluffier'.

Scatter the tomatoes over the egg and cook for 2 minutes or until just set. Crumble or grate the cheese over the top, fold the omelette in half and slide straight onto a warmed plate. Eat immediately, ideally with a lightly dressed salad.

Apple pancakes with blueberries and banana

Lovely and light, with a great burst of flavour, these fluffy pancakes contain grated apple for a prebiotic boost. Use an extra 25ml of milk if you make the pancakes with self-raising brown flour.

SERVES 2 | **PREP:** 5 minutes | **COOK:** 10 minutes

100g self-raising white flour or self-raising brown or wholemeal flour
¼ tsp ground cinnamon (optional)
1 large egg
125ml semi-skimmed or whole milk
1 eating apple
1 tsp extra virgin olive oil
50g fresh blueberries

1 just-ripe banana, peeled and sliced
25g pecan nuts or mixed nuts, roughly chopped
runny honey or maple syrup and full-fat live natural yogurt, to serve

Put the flour and cinnamon in a bowl, make a well in the centre and break the egg into it. Using a metal whisk, beat the egg and half the milk to form a thick batter. Add all the remaining milk and beat hard until the batter is as smooth and lump-free as possible.

Coarsely grate the apple, including the skin, onto a board, avoiding the core. Stir the grated apple into the pancake batter.

Brush a large non-stick frying pan with the oil and place over a medium heat. Spoon a quarter of the batter into one side of the pan and spread gently with the back of a spoon. Make a second pancake in the same way. Cook both pancakes together for 2 minutes or until small bubbles appear on the surface of each pancake and the tops are beginning to set, then carefully flip over and cook on the other side for 1½–2 minutes more.

Transfer the pancakes to a warmed plate and cook the remaining 2 pancakes in exactly the same way.

Divide the pancakes between two warmed plates and top with blueberries, sliced bananas and pecan nuts. Drizzle with the honey or maple syrup and serve hot with spoonfuls of yogurt.

Lower-sugar plum freezer jam

I love serving this fruit-heavy, very softly set jam with spoonfuls of homemade Yogurt cheese (see page 246) and toasted sourdough or wholegrain bread for a lazy weekend breakfast. It has a lot less sugar than traditional jam, so won't keep as long without freezing. Divided into small pots and use when needed.

SERVES 8 | **PREP:** 10 minutes, plus standing
COOK: 20–25 minutes

400g fresh plums, stoned and
   quartered
4 tbsp cold water
65g jam sugar (with added pectin)

Put the plums in a saucepan and add the water. Cover with a lid and cook over a low heat for 15 minutes, removing the lid and stirring occasionally until very soft.

Add the jam sugar and stir for about a minute or until the sugar has dissolved. Increase the heat and boil for about 8 minutes, stirring regularly until the jam is thickened and glossy.

Once the jam is cold, divide between two small lidded containers. Put one in the fridge to use within 3 days and freeze the rest for up to three months. Take out of the freezer as you need them and thaw overnight in the fridge. Stir well before using.

COOK'S TIP
Making my own jam means I can pick really good prebiotic fruits and keep the sugar levels as low as possible. This one uses fresh plums and jam sugar with added pectin – a recognised prebiotic. Pectin is made from crushed apples in the UK and helps guarantee a good set for any jams and marmalades. And who knows, even in tiny quantities like this, it could bestow some prebiotic benefits at breakfast. You'll find this in the same aisle as the other sugars and online. If you can't get hold of it, use any white sugar.

Yogurt cheese

This tangy spread isn't really a cheese at all but probiotic yogurt with a high proportion of the whey (watery liquid) strained out overnight. It's a good addition to your recipe repertoire as it's guaranteed to contain probiotic bacteria – as long as you choose a good-quality live yogurt. You will need to get hold of some muslin to make it – look in cookshops and online – although I have heard of people straining their yogurt through a brand-new J-cloth too. If you start off with Greek yogurt that's already been strained to some extent, you'll end up with a firmer 'cheese'.

SERVES 2 | **PREP:** 5 minutes, plus overnight

200g full-fat live natural yogurt

Line sieve with a square of muslin and place over a small bowl. Spoon the yogurt into the bowl, then pull up the ends of the muslin and tie together to enclose the yogurt.

Place in the fridge overnight to strain. Discard the liquid and transfer the yogurt 'cheese' to a small dish. Cover, keep in the fridge and eat within 3 days.

MAKE A CHANGE
To make a probiotic garlic and herb cheese to serve with a gut-happy platter, mix the soft 'cheese' with 1 crushed garlic clove, 1 teaspoon finely chopped fresh parsley, 1 teaspoon finely chopped fresh chives and a pinch of salt.

Ten-plus salads

A really good mixed salad can contain a variety of prebiotic and probiotic ingredients. If you aim for at least five different plant-based ingredients for a salad to serve alongside another dish and around ten different ingredients for a main meal salad, you can be pretty sure that you are treating your gut microbes to a feast. Even small amounts of extra virgin olive oil in a dressing count and, amazingly enough, adding fat to green leaves actually makes the nutrients easier to absorb too.

That sort of flexibility should make it simpler for you to stick to the plan. If there are days that you really don't have time to prepare or cook a salad from scratch, simply buy a ready-made one from a supermarket, cafe, restaurant or delicatessen. Try to pick salads with lots of different vegetables, beans or lentils, wholegrains, nuts and seeds. Avoid any with thick mayonnaise-style dressings and those with only five main ingredients or fewer if possible.

You don't need a huge amount as your bowl will be quickly filled with all these colourful combinations. And, of course, feel free to add any other vegetables or fruit – depending on where you live, you may find much more variety with unusual, more exotic imported ingredients widely available in your area. If you do try something different, don't forget to jot it down in your journal.

For the Ten-plus salad recipes in this chapter, I've tried to ensure a good range of different colours, textures and flavours. They mainly serve two people, but a few stretch to four and can be served over a couple of days if you like. If you are planning to take to work, do all the preparation the night before then assemble the salad in the morning, packing into lidded containers or wide-mouthed sturdy jars. Keep chilled until you are ready to serve.

The recipes

Greek-plus salad

Pear, barley, blue cheese and pecan salad

Quinoa, sweetcorn, avocado and chilli salad

Salmon rice salad

Tuna and mixed bean salad

Blushing roots and soft cheese salad

Roast sweet potato, quinoa and lentil salad

Chicken noodle salad

Spiced chicken and rice salad

Greek-plus salad

This Greek-style salad has the addition of artichoke hearts and butterbeans to give it extra fermentable fibre. Add the leftover beans to soups, stews and curries or serve tossed with a garlicky vinaigrette or fresh pesto as part of a gut-happy platter the next day.

SERVES 2 | **PREP:** 15 minutes

½ small red onion, peeled
2 large ripe tomatoes
sea salt and black pepper
½ cucumber (about 200g)
100g feta cheese, drained and cut into small cubes
50g pitted black olives (preferably Kalamata), drained

4 chargrilled artichoke hearts (from a tub or jar), drained and quartered
½ 400g can butterbeans or cannellini beans, rinsed and drained
small handful fresh mint leaves
½ tsp dried oregano
2 tbsp extra virgin olive oil
2 tsp fresh lemon juice

Slice the onion very thinly and put into a medium bowl. Cut the tomatoes into chunky pieces and add to the bowl with the onion. Season well with salt and pepper.

Cut the cucumber in half lengthways and scoop out the seeds with a teaspoon, if you like. Thickly slice the cucumber and add to the onion and tomatoes.

Scatter the feta, olives, artichokes, beans and mint leaves on top. Sprinkle over the oregano and toss lightly together. Drizzle over the oil and lemon juice and serve.

Pear, barley, blue cheese and pecan salad

A fresh-tasting, fruity salad with added prebiotic pearl barley and artichokes and some microbe-enhancing unpasteurised (raw milk) cheese.

SERVES 2–3 | **PREP:** 20 minutes

50g pearl barley

25g mixed salad leaves, such as endive, radicchio and lamb's lettuce

1 red or white chicory, trimmed and thickly sliced

1 firm but ripe pear, quartered, cored and sliced

4 chargrilled artichoke hearts (from a jar or tub), drained and quartered

35g unpasteurised (raw) blue cheese, such as Roquefort or Stilton

25g shelled pecan nuts, walnuts or mixed nuts, roughly chopped

2 spring onions, trimmed and thinly sliced

sea salt and black pepper

For the vinaigrette:

1 tsp Dijon mustard

1 tsp caster sugar (optional)

2 tsp red wine vinegar or cider vinegar

½ small garlic clove, peeled and crushed

salt and black pepper

4 tbsp extra virgin olive oil

Half-fill a medium saucepan with water and stir in the pearl barley. Bring to the boil and cook for about 25 minutes, or until tender, stirring occasionally. Drain in a sieve under running water until cold.

Make the vinaigrette. Put the mustard, sugar, if using, vinegar and crushed garlic in a bowl and season with a pinch of salt and some ground black pepper. Whisk with a metal whisk until well combined. Gradually add the oil, whisking constantly until the dressing is thick. Adjust the seasoning to taste.

Shake the salad leaves onto a platter and top with the cooked barley, chicory, pear and artichoke. Break the cheese into pieces with your fingers and drop gently on top. Scatter the nuts and spring onion over, drizzle with the dressing and serve immediately.

Cook an extra 25g pearl barley in the same pan so you have it ready to use for a salad the next day. Once drained and rinsed, put in a covered bowl in the fridge until needed.

Quinoa, sweetcorn, avocado and chilli salad

The dressing for this salad gets its smoky flavour from chipotle paste, made from smoked jalapeño peppers. You can find it in the Mexican section of larger supermarkets. Alternatively, add a teaspoon of hot smoked paprika to the dressing. Quinoa is a highly nutritious South American seed that can be served in a similar way to rice.

SERVES 4 | **PREP:** 20 minutes | **COOK:** 12 minutes

75g uncooked quinoa (a mix of red and white is nice - or combined with bulgur)

198g can sweetcorn, drained, or 100g frozen sweetcorn, thawed

400g can red kidney beans, rinsed and drained

100g cherry tomatoes, halved

bunch coriander, leaves roughly chopped

3 spring onions, trimmed and finely sliced

½ long red chilli, finely chopped (deseeded first if you like)

2 ripe but firm avocados, stoned, peeled and sliced

100g bag mixed salad leaves

2 tbsp mixed seeds, such as sunflower, pumpkin, linseed and sesame

sea salt and black pepper

For the dressing:

fresh juice of 1 lime (you need roughly 2 tbsp lime juice)

1–2 tsp chipotle paste (from a jar)

1 garlic clove, peeled and crushed

2 tbsp extra virgin olive oil

sea salt and black pepper

Fill a medium saucepan a third of the way with water and bring to the boil. Rinse the quinoa in a fine sieve then add to the water, stir well and simmer for about 12 minutes, or until just tender. It is ready when it begins to shed the 'c'-shaped outer husks.

Rinse the cooked quinoa in a sieve under cold water, then press hard with a ladle or serving spoon to remove as much of the excess water as possible.

Tip the quinoa into a bowl and toss with the dressing ingredients, sweetcorn, kidney beans, tomatoes, coriander, spring onions and chilli. Season well with salt and pepper. It's important to make sure that the dressing is mixed well through the salad.

Add the avocados and leaves to the salad and toss gently together. Sprinkle with mixed seeds and serve.

TIME-SAVING TIP
If making this recipe for two people, divide the salad in half after tossing with the dressing. Add one of the avocados and half the leaves to one portion and cover and chill the other in the fridge ready to eat the next day. Slice the remaining avocado and add to the salad along with the mixed leaves and seeds just before serving.

Salmon rice salad

A zingy salad that makes a wonderful fresh-tasting packed lunch. Keep the dressing separate in a small jar and drizzle over the salad just before serving. To serve warm, reheat the rice, broccoli and salmon in the microwave then spoon over the dressing.

SERVES 2 | **PREP:** 15 minutes | **COOK:** 20 minutes

100g mixed basmati and wild rice

100g long tender stem broccoli, cut into short lengths

25g cashew nuts, lightly toasted (if liked) and roughly chopped

bunch fresh coriander, leaves roughly chopped (optional)

2 little gem lettuces, separated into leaves

150g cooked salmon

lime wedges, to serve

For the dressing:

juice of 1 small lime (about 2 tbsp)

1 tsp runny honey

1 tbsp dark soy sauce

sea salt and black pepper

2 tbsp extra virgin olive oil

Half-fill a medium saucepan with water and bring to the boil. Put the rice in a sieve and rinse under plenty of cold water – this will remove the excess starch and help keep the grains separate as they cook.

Add the rice to the water, stir well and return to the boil. Cook for 20–25 minutes or until just tender. Add the broccoli and cook with the rice for 2–3 minutes more or until the broccoli is tender, stirring occasionally.

While the rice is cooking, make the dressing. Pour the lime juice into a bowl – you should have 2 tablespoons of lime juice – and whisk in the honey, soy sauce, a good pinch of salt and some ground black pepper. Slowly whisk in the oil until the dressing is slightly thickened.

Drain the rice and broccoli in a sieve under running water until cold and tip into the bowl with the dressing, add the nuts and coriander and toss well together.

Divide the lettuce leaves between two bowls or containers. Divide the rice salad between the bowls and add the salmon, flaked into chunky pieces. Serve with extra lime wedges and coriander for garnishing if you like.

TIME-SAVING TIP

To make it easier, you can buy roasted salmon from the chiller cabinet – the kind that is lightly smoked too if you can find it. Otherwise, bake a couple of salmon fillets on a baking tray in a preheated oven at 200°C/fan oven 180°C/gas 6 for about 15 minutes and leave to cool before flaking on top of the salad.

MAKE A CHANGE

Use leftover cold cooked chicken for this salad if you like, or make meat-free by adding lightly stir-fried vegetables.

Tuna and mixed bean salad

Layered salads are great for packed lunches and picnics. You need to make sure the dressing is kept at the bottom of the dish and then the salad mixed just before serving or it could go soggy. Make in one large bowl if you are eating at home, or divide between two sturdy containers if you are taking to work. This salad makes two generous portions.

SERVES 2–3 | **PREP:** 10 minutes

1 tsp Dijon mustard
1 tsp caster sugar
1 small garlic clove, crushed
1 tbsp white wine vinegar
4 tbsp extra virgin olive oil
sea salt and black pepper
400g can mixed beans, drained and rinsed
½ small red onion, finely sliced

1 medium carrot, peeled and coarsely grated
8 cherry tomatoes, halved
50g crispy leaf salad, containing a mixture of curly endive, radicchio and lamb's lettuce
198g can tuna steak in spring water, drained

Put the mustard, sugar, garlic, vinegar and oil in a bowl, add a pinch of salt and some ground black pepper and whisk with a small metal whisk until slightly thickened.

Add the beans to the bowl and stir in the red onion. Place the carrot, tomatoes and mixed salad on top without stirring.

With a fork, flake the tuna out of the can and onto the salad. Season with ground black pepper. Cover and keep chilled until ready to serve, then lightly toss all the ingredients.

Blushing roots and soft cheese salad

This easy roasted vegetable recipe is packed with naturally sweet vegetables to help keep sugar cravings at bay. You can press the softened garlic cloves out of their skins and mash with the roasted vegetables as you eat the salad. I've called it blushing roots as the juice from the beetroot leaches out as it softens and gives a pinky blush to the rest of the vegetables.

SERVES 2 | **PREP:** 30 minutes | **COOK:** 1 hour

½ small butternut squash (about 350g), peeled deseeded, and cut into roughly 2cm chunks

1 medium carrot, cut into roughly 2cm chunks

1 small parsnip (about 125g), peeled and cut into roughly 2cm chunks

1 raw beetroot (about 200g), well scrubbed and cut into thick wedges

2 tbsp extra virgin olive oil, plus 1 tbsp for drizzling

juice and finely grated zest of 1 lemon

salt and pepper

8 garlic cloves, unpeeled

4–5 sprigs thyme, leaves roughly chopped (you'll need 1 tbsp leaves)

50g mixed nuts, such as Brazils, almonds, hazelnuts, pecans and walnuts, roughly chopped

25g mixed baby leaves, such as watercress, rocket and spinach

100g soft cheese ideally unpasteurised (raw milk), such as goat's cheese, or homemade Yogurt cheese (page 246)

2–3 tsp good-quality balsamic vinegar

Heat oven to 200°C/fan oven 180°C /gas 6. Put the vegetables, without the garlic, into a bowl and toss with 2 tablespoons of the oil, lemon juice and zest and plenty of ground black pepper. Scatter the vegetables over a large baking tray or roasting tin and bake for 20 minutes.

Take the tray out of the oven, add the garlic and thyme and turn the vegetables. Return to the oven for another 20 minutes. Remove the tray once more, sprinkle with the nuts and return to the oven for a further 10 minutes or until the vegetables are tender and lightly browned.

Divide the leaves between 2 deep plates and top with the warm vegetables, dot with small knobs of the cheese and drizzle with the remaining olive oil and a splash of balsamic vinegar.

COOK'S TIP

It's not absolutely essential to peel the squash, just make sure you wash it very well before roasting. Either eat the baked skin or scrape the flesh off the skin once served.

Roast sweet potato, quinoa and lentil salad

This is one of my favourite salads and it always makes an appearance at family parties in our house. It has a lot of different elements but is very easy to prepare and the combination of flavours and textures is incredibly delicious.

SERVES 4 | **PREP:** 25 minutes | **COOK:** 30–40 minutes

1 large sweet potato (about 300g), cut into roughly 3cm chunks

2 tbsp extra virgin olive oil

1 red pepper, deseeded and cut into roughly 3cm chunks

1 yellow or orange pepper, deseeded and cut into roughly 3cm chunks

40g quinoa (a mix of red and white is nice)

75g uncooked bulgur wheat

75g dried puy or green lentils, rinsed in cold water and drained

1 medium carrot, finely diced

finely grated zest of 1 lemon

4 spring onions, trimmed and finely sliced

50g small bag of baby salad leaves, such as watercress, spinach and rocket

sea salt and black pepper

For the dressing:

1 tsp Dijon mustard

1 tsp caster sugar

1 tbsp red wine or cider vinegar

1 small garlic clove, crushed

sea salt and black pepper

5 tbsp extra virgin olive oil

Preheat the oven to 200°C/fan oven 180°C/gas 6. Put the sweet potato in a bowl and toss with 1 tablespoon of the oil. Scatter over a baking tray and season with salt and pepper. Bake for 10 minutes, then add the peppers and mix lightly. Return to the oven for a further 20 minutes or until the vegetables are tender and lightly browned.

Half-fill 2 medium saucepans with water and bring to the boil. Cook the lentils for 25–35 minutes in one pan and the quinoa and bulgur in a different pan for about 10 minutes or until tender. The quinoa is ready when the 'c'-shaped husks just begin to separate from the seeds.

Drain then rinse the quinoa and bulgur in a sieve under running water until cold. Drain well and press with the back of a spoon to get rid of as much water as possible. Tip into a large mixing bowl. Drain the puy lentils and rinse under running water until cold. Drain and add to the bowl.

Take the sweet potato and peppers out of the oven and leave to cool.

To make the dressing, put the mustard, sugar, vinegar and crushed garlic in a bowl and season with a pinch of salt and some ground black pepper. Whisk with a small metal whisk until well combined. Gradually add the oil, whisking constantly until the dressing is thick. Adjust the seasoning to taste. (Taste, and add a little more olive oil if necessary.)

To assemble the salad, add the carrot, lemon zest, spring onions, peppers and sweet potatoes to the lentils, quinoa and bulgur. Season with salt and pepper. Toss well together. (This can be done up to 8 hours ahead, covered and kept in the fridge.)

Just before serving, add the baby salad leaves, give the dressing a quick whisk to re-emulsify, pour the dressing over and toss lightly together.

Chicken noodle salad

Cold noodle salads make great packed lunches and this one can be made a day ahead and will still taste fabulous. Look out for packets of frozen edamame/soya beans (without their pods) as they make an interesting and delicious change from peas, or use frozen baby broad beans instead.

SERVES 4 | **PREP:** 15 minutes | **COOK:** 20 minutes, plus standing

2 boneless, skinless chicken breasts (each about 150g)
½ tsp ground ginger
2 tbsp dark soy sauce
100g wholewheat egg noodles
2 large carrots
100g mangetout or sugar snap peas, trimmed and halved lengthways
100g frozen edamame beans or frozen peas
6 spring onions, trimmed and finely sliced

1 tsp sesame seeds or 1 tbsp mixed seeds
sea salt and black pepper

For the dressing:
2 tbsp caster sugar
6 tbsp cold water
1-2 tsp red chilli paste (from a jar), or 1 plump red chilli, deseeded and finely chopped
1 tbsp dark soy sauce
2 tsp toasted sesame oil

To make the dressing, put the sugar in a small saucepan with the water and heat gently until dissolved. Bring to the boil and cook for 1 minute, stirring. Take off the heat and stir in the chilli paste, soy sauce and sesame oil. Tip into a heatproof bowl and leave to cool.

Preheat the oven to 210°C/fan oven 190°C/gas 6½. Put the chicken in a small ovenproof dish or tin and rub with the ginger. Brush with the soy sauce and season with black pepper. Bake for 15-18 minutes or until cooked through and lightly browned. Put on a board and rest for 10 minutes.

While the chicken is cooking, half-fill a saucepan with water and bring to the boil. Add the noodles and cook for 3 minutes, or according to the packet instructions, until tender, stirring occasionally to separate the strands. Drain in a colander and rinse under running water until cold. Tip into a large mixing bowl.

Peel the carrots and cut into long, thin strips. Place the strips in a pile on top of each other. (You can also coarsely grate the carrots if you prefer.) Add the carrots, mangetout and edamame beans or frozen peas to the salad (there is no need to thaw them first).

Slice the chicken widthways and add to the noodles and vegetables. Pour over the dressing and toss well together.
Add the spring onions and sesame seeds and toss lightly. Stand for 5 minutes before serving or cover and chill. Eat within 2 days.

TIME-SAVING TIP

Red chilli paste is a useful ingredient to have in the fridge and can be stirred into all sorts of dressings and sauces. It also saves the bother of chopping up fresh chillies and you can adjust the heat to suit yourself.

MAKE A CHANGE

You can serve this salad hot if you like. Simply transfer to a suitable bowl and reheat in the microwave for 3–4 minutes, stirring halfway through the cooking time.

Spiced chicken and rice salad

This is a great salad for a summer lunch and a brilliant dish for a packed lunch. Keep cool until you are ready to eat.

SERVES 3 | **PREP:** 15 minutes, plus chilling | **COOK:** 25 minutes

1 tbsp extra virgin olive oil

1 medium red onion, peeled and finely chopped

1 yellow or orange pepper, deseeded and cut into roughly 2cm chunks

100g broccoli, cut into small florets and halved

100g easy-cook wholegrain or brown rice (such as Uncle Ben's)

2 tsp medium curry powder

100g cooked and cooled skinless chicken meat

100g red seedless grapes, halved

½ cucumber (about 100g), cut into small chunks

25g toasted flaked almonds

bunch fresh coriander, leaves roughly chopped

For the dressing:

1 tbsp fresh lime juice

1 tsp caster sugar

1 tsp medium curry powder

1 garlic clove, peeled and crushed

sea salt and black pepper

3 tbsp extra virgin olive oil

Heat the oil in a large non-stick frying pan and gently fry the onion, pepper and broccoli for 4–5 minutes, stirring occasionally until the vegetables are softened but still retain some 'bite'. Remove from the heat and spread onto a plate, to cool.

Half-fill a pan with water and bring to the boil. Stir in the rice and the curry powder. Return to the boil and cook for 10–15 minutes or until tender, stirring occasionally. Drain in a sieve and rinse under running water until cold. Drain well and transfer to a large bowl. Cut the chicken into bite-sized pieces and add to the rice. Stir in the cooled vegetables, grapes, cucumber, almonds and coriander.

Make the dressing by whisking the lime juice, sugar, curry powder and garlic together with a little salt and lots of ground black pepper. Gradually whisk in the olive oil. Pour over the salad and toss well together. Keep chilled until ready to serve.

Salsas, small salads and sides

One of the best ways to increase your intake of fibre and polyphenol-rich ingredients is to add a serving of a salsa or relish, salad or other accompaniment to your main meals.

By using recipes in this section, it's easy to make dishes you already cook regularly, and feel confident serving, that bit more gut-healthy. And these recipes crop up regularly in the 28-day plan too.

I've included lots of polyphenol-rich olive oil and nuts, plus side dishes containing vegetables and pulses to introduce extra prebiotic fibre that should help keep your gut microbes well nourished.

The recipes

Fresh tomato salsa

Zingy avocado salsa

Minted yogurt and cucumber

Simple gut-happy salad

Rainbow coleslaw

Leftover potato salad

Mexican rice salad

Lunchbox salad

Five-plus mixed veg

Easy roasted vegetables

Broccoli and almond rice

Celeriac mash

Spinach and potato mash

Simple vegetable stir-fry

Bulgur wheat salad

Warm beans with garlic and lemon

Fresh tomato salsa

A fab fresh relish that features inulin-rich garlic and onion, and is perfect served alongside all sorts of hot foods. Try with curries, chilli and grilled meat or fish for a burst of extra vitamins and polyphenols. It's also great as part of a gut-happy platter or stuffed into wholemeal wraps with stir-fried chicken strips, peppers and onions, plus spoonfuls of full-fat live natural yogurt, for a healthier fajita or lunchtime wrap.

SERVES 4 | **PREP:** 10 minutes

- 1 small red onion, peeled, quartered and finely sliced
- 1 large garlic clove, peeled and crushed
- 2 medium ripe tomatoes (about 200g), roughly chopped
- bunch fresh coriander, leaves roughly chopped
- 1 red or green chilli, deseeded and finely chopped (optional)
- 1 tbsp extra virgin olive oil
- sea salt and black pepper

Mix the onion, garlic, tomatoes, coriander leaves, chilli and oil. Season with salt and pepper. Leave to stand for 10 minutes before serving.

TIME-SAVING TIP
This salsa keeps well for a couple of days in the fridge. Simply put into a small bowl and cover tightly.

Zingy avocado salsa

A great topping for spicy dishes, such as my Smoky bean chilli
or Lamb and sweet potato tagine, or it can be rolled into wraps,
spread onto wholegrain toast or mashed for a quick dip. Serve as
part of a gut-happy platter too if you like.

SERVES 4 | **PREP:** 5 minutes

1 ripe but firm avocado
freshly squeezed juice of 1 lime
2 spring onions, trimmed and finely
  sliced
1 garlic clove, peeled and crushed
sea salt and black pepper

Cut the avocado in half and remove the stone. Slide a large metal
spoon around each half of the avocado to scoop out the flesh.

Cut into small pieces and toss with the lime juice, garlic and
spring onions; season with salt and pepper and toss well together.

Minted yogurt and cucumber

SERVES 2 | **PREP:** 5 minutes

150g full-fat live natural yogurt
1 tbsp finely chopped fresh mint
   leaves
¼ large cucumber (about 100g),
   diced

Put the yogurt in a small bowl and stir in the mint and cucumber.
Season with a good pinch of salt and some ground black pepper.

COOK'S TIP
Add a few tablespoons of milk kefir to this tangy dip if you have
some handy.

Simple gut-happy salad

A good basic salad containing gut-friendly onion, beans, olive oil and nuts, as well as vitamin-rich leaves and tomatoes.

SERVES 2 | **PREP:** 10 minutes

2 ripe tomatoes, cut into quarters
1 small red onion, peeled and very thinly sliced
120g canned haricot beans (½ a 400g can), drained and rinsed
1 red or white chicory, trimmed and thickly sliced
25g mixed nuts, roughly chopped
25g (2 handfuls) mixed spinach, watercress and rocket salad

1 tbsp mixed seeds, such as sunflowers, pumpkin linseed (flax) and sesame

For the French dressing:
1 tsp Dijon mustard
½ tsp golden caster sugar
1 tsp red wine or cider vinegar
½ garlic clove, peeled and crushed
3 tbsp extra virgin olive oil
sea salt and ground black pepper

Toss all the salad ingredients lightly in a serving bowl.

Whisk together the mustard, sugar, vinegar, garlic, a pinch of salt and lots of ground black pepper in a small bowl. Gradually add the olive oil, whisking until well combined, thickened and glossy.

Drizzle the dressing over the salad. Sprinkle with seeds and serve.

MAKE A CHANGE
Use any cooked beans you like for this salad. If taking from a 400g can, rinse in a sieve under running water then use half for the salad. Put the rest in a bowl and toss lightly with 2 teaspoons of extra virgin olive oil. Cover and keep in the fridge. Eat within two days.

Rainbow coleslaw

A great coleslaw to serve alongside grilled and pan-fried meats and fish. It also goes extremely well with my Beany nut burgers (page 218). Grapes and nuts contain known gut-healthy polyphenols and red cabbage contains anti-inflammatory polyphenols called anthocyanins.

SERVES 2-3 | **PREP:** 10 minutes

2 tbsp extra virgin olive oil
2 tsp fresh lemon juice
sea salt and black pepper
150g red cabbage (about ¼ small red cabbage)
1 medium carrot
1 medium eating apple, quartered, cored and cut into small chunks

75g seedless red grapes, halved
2 spring onions, trimmed and finely sliced, including lots of green
25g sultanas or raisins
25g mixed nuts, roughly chopped
2 tbsp mixed seeds, such as sunflower, pumpkin, sesame and linseed

Whisk the oil and lemon juice together in a large bowl with a metal whisk and season with lots of ground black pepper.

Remove any damaged outer leaves from the cabbage, cut out the white core and finely slice the leaves without separating. The finer you can slice, the easier it will be to eat the coleslaw.

Coarsely grate the carrot, carefully holding it almost vertically against the grater so you get nice long strands – watch your fingers towards the end.

Add the cabbage, carrot, apple, grapes, spring onions, sultanas, nuts and seeds to the dressing and toss well together.

COOK'S TIP
Slice the cabbage from root end to tip to help keep the leaves nice and fine, but don't worry if a few of them are a bit chunkier. Cover any remaining cabbage tightly with cling film and use for mixed salads and for serving alongside main meal dishes. You can also brine-pickled red cabbage to produce lots of probiotic bacteria.

Leftover potato salad

Make this simple salad for lunch using potatoes leftover from
dinner the night before. Because the potatoes have been cooked
and cooled, they will contain more microbe-friendly resistant
starch and be healthier.

SERVES 2 | **PREP:** 5 minutes

150g cooked and cooled new
  potatoes, thickly sliced
1 red eating apple, quartered, cored
  and cut into small chunks
1 celery stick, trimmed and thinly
  sliced

25g mixed nuts, roughly chopped
1 spring onion or a small handful
  fresh chives, finely sliced
Olive oil vinaigrette (page 292)

Put the potatoes, apples, celery, nuts and spring onions or chives
in a bowl. Add 2 tbsp Olive oil vinaigrette and mix lightly.
  Divide the salad between two serving bowls or lidded containers.
Cover and keep in the fridge if not serving immediately. Toss
lightly just before serving.

MAKE A CHANGE
You can make a probiotic dressing for this salad by mixing 1 tbsp
of the Olive oil vinaigrette with 4 tbsp full-fat live natural yogurt or
milk kefir instead.

Mexican rice salad

Make this fibre-rich salad for lunch using rice leftover from
dinner the night before. Cook double what you need then divide
the portions and make sure you cool your salad rice quickly –
rinsing in cold water is a good idea. Put into a lidded container
and keep chilled until you are ready to serve.

SERVES 2 | **PREP:** 15 minutes

150g cooked and cooled mixed rice
(see tip below)
50g frozen sweetcorn, thawed
½ red pepper, deseeded and diced
fresh coriander, leaves roughly
chopped
½ ripe avocado, stoned, peeled and
diced

For the dressing:
2 tbsp fresh lime juice
1 tbsp runny honey
½ tsp chipotle paste (from a jar)
1 small garlic clove, peeled and
crushed
3 tbsp extra virgin olive oil
sea salt and black pepper

Put the rice, sweetcorn, pepper and coriander in a bowl and mix
together lightly.

Put the dressing ingredients in a bowl and whisk with a metal
whisk until slightly thickened. Season with salt and pepper.

Divide the salad between two serving bowls or lidded containers
and scatter the avocado on top. Spoon over the dressing, making
sure it covers the cut surfaces of the avocado.

Cover and keep in the fridge if not serving immediately. Toss the
salad lightly just before serving.

TIME-SAVING TIP
You can make the dressing ahead of time but it is best to eat
the salad the same day it is made and before the avocado has a
chance to turn brown.

MAKE A CHANGE

To make 150g cold cooked rice, you will need to start with 75g mixed rice. I use one that contains brown basmati rice, red rice and wild rice but you can use a plain wholegrain rice if you prefer. Half-fill a medium pan with water and bring to the boil. Add the rice and cook for 25–35 minutes or until tender, stirring occasionally. Drain in a sieve and rinse under running water until cold.

Lunchbox salad

This delicious salad mixes wholegrain rice, lentils and barley with lots of fresh vegetables and herbs.

SERVES 2 | **PREP:** 15 minutes

40g cooked and cooled wholegrain rice

25g cooked and cooled puy or green lentils

25g cooked and cooled pearl barley

1 red or white chicory, trimmed and leaves separated

150g cherry tomatoes (about 16), halved

4 radishes, finely sliced

bunch fresh parsley, leaves roughly chopped

2 spring onions, trimmed and finely sliced

25g mixed nuts, roughly chopped

For the dressing:

4 tbsp olive oil vinaigrette (page 292)

Put the rice, lentils, barley, tomatoes, radishes and parsley in a bowl and mix lightly.

Divide between two serving bowls or lidded containers. Cover and keep in the fridge if not serving immediately. Just before serving, spoon over the dressing and toss lightly.

MAKE A CHANGE

To make the salad using uncooked wholegrains, half-fill a large pan with water and bring to the boil. Add the rice, lentils and pearl barley and return to the boil. Cook for 25–35 minutes or until tender, stirring occasionally. Drain in a sieve and rinse under running water until cold. If using easy-cook wholegrain rice, cook separately for 10 minutes or according to the packet instructions.

Five-plus mixed veg

This is a great mix of vegetables to serve alongside almost anything. They are all cooked in one pan, saving you lots of space on the hob, and it only takes a few minutes to make. Feel free to swap other vegetables of your choice with my suggestions, but keep the total number of vegetables up to five or more if you can.

SERVES 2 | **PREP:** 5 minutes | **COOK:** 10 minutes

1 medium carrot, thinly sliced

1 slender leek, trimmed and cut into roughly 1cm slices

4 asparagus spears or long-stemmed broccoli, trimmed and halved

1 small courgette, halved lengthways and cut into roughly 1cm slices

50g frozen peas

1 tbsp extra virgin olive oil or small knob of butter

sea salt and black pepper

Half fill a medium saucepan with water and bring to the boil. Add the carrot and cook for 5 minutes, stirring occasionally.

Next, add the leek, asparagus or broccoli, courgette and peas. Return the water to the boil and cook for 2–3 minutes more, or until all the vegetables are just tender.

Drain in a colander then place in a warmed serving dish, drizzle with the oil (or dot with the butter) and toss lightly. Season with ground black pepper and serve.

COOK'S TIP

If you are using fairly thick asparagus rather than fine spears, you'll need to add it at the same time as the carrot or it won't be tender. Toss the cooked vegetables with finely chopped fresh herbs if you like.

Easy roasted vegetables

A simple selection of vegetables that you can bung in the oven and forget about while you get on with other things. Use any leftover vegetables for a gut-happy platter or salad the next day.

SERVES 2 | **PREP:** 10 minutes | **COOK:** 40 minutes

1 red pepper, deseeded and cut into roughly 2cm chunks

1 yellow pepper, deseeded and cut into roughly 2cm chunks

1 medium sweet potato (about 300g), cut into roughly 2cm chunks

1 medium courgette, cut in half lengthways and then into roughly 1.5cm slices

1 medium red onion, cut into 10 thin wedges

2 tbsp extra virgin olive oil, plus extra for drizzling

8 garlic cloves (unpeeled)

½ tsp dried chilli flakes (optional)

sea salt and black pepper

Preheat the oven to 220°C/fan oven 200°C/gas 7. Put all the vegetables in a large bowl and toss with the oil. Season with a large pinch of salt and lots of ground black pepper. Scatter over a baking tray in a single layer and roast for 10 minutes.

Take the baking tray out of the oven, scatter with the garlic and sprinkle with the chilli flakes, if using. Turn all the vegetables and return to the oven for a further 20 minutes, or until all the vegetables are nicely browned and the garlic is tender.

Squeeze the garlic purée out of the skins as you eat it. (Don't eat the papery skins.)

Broccoli and almond rice

A great way of adding extra gut-happy ingredients to your meal.
Choose a pack of rice that includes at least one wholegrain.
You can also make this dish using brown rice and quinoa mixes.
If you don't have flaked almonds to hand, use any mix of nuts,
roughly chopped, instead.

SERVES 2 | **PREP:** 5 minutes | **COOK:** 25–30 minutes

100g ready-mixed rice, such as
brown basmati, red Camargue
and wild rice, or any wholegrain
rice

75g long-stemmed broccoli
25g toasted flaked almonds

Half-fill a medium saucepan with cold water and add the rice.
Bring to the boil, stirring occasionally, then loosely cover and cook
for 22–28 minutes, or according to the packet instructions, until
tender. Remove the lid every now and then and give it a quick stir.
   Trim the broccoli, cut into roughly 2cm lengths and add to the
boiling water. Return to the boil and cook for 2 minutes more or
until just tender. Drain the broccoli and rice well and toss with the
flaked almonds.

MAKE A CHANGE
If you can't get hold of toasted almonds, put plain flaked almonds
into a non-stick frying pan and toast over a medium heat for
3–5 minutes, turning occasionally.

Celeriac mash

Cooking celeriac with potatoes adds an extra vegetable to your meal. This creamy tasting mash goes extremely well with any roasted or grilled meat or fish.

SERVES 2 | **PREP:** 20 minutes | **COOK:** 15–20 minutes

400g medium floury potatoes (preferably Maris Piper or King Edwards), peeled and cut into roughly 4cm chunks

½ large celeriac (about 340g), peeled and cut into 4cm chunks

25g butter
50ml semi-skimmed or whole milk
1 garlic clove, peeled and crushed
a good pinch ground nutmeg
sea salt and black pepper

Put the potatoes and celeriac into a large pan and cover with cold water. Bring to a simmer, cover loosely with a lid and cook for about 20 minutes or until both vegetables are very tender. Drain in a colander and leave to stand for a couple of minutes before returning to the pan.

While the vegetables are standing, warm the butter and milk in a small saucepan with the garlic and nutmeg until the butter melts.

Pour the warm milk over the potatoes, season with a little salt and lots of ground black pepper. Mash well until as smooth as possible. Adjust seasoning to taste.

FREEZING TIP

Flat-freeze cooked and cooled leftover mash in small freezer-proof containers for up to two months. Thaw overnight in the fridge then reheat in the microwave, or a wide-based pan over a medium heat, stirring regularly until hot throughout.

MAKE A CHANGE

If you are cooking roast pork, make an apple mash by simmering chopped, peeled cooking apple with the celeriac and potatoes for additional prebiotic fibre.

Spinach and potato mash

SERVES 4 | **PREP:** 25 minutes | **COOK:** 15 minutes

750g medium floury potatoes,
   (preferably Maris Piper or King
   Edward), peeled and cut into
   roughly 4–5cm chunks
2 tbsp extra virgin olive oil, plus
   extra fro drizzling
100g young spinach leaves
1 garlic clove, peeled and crushed
6 spring onions, trimmed and finely
   sliced
40g butter
100ml semi-skimmed or whole milk
100g full-fat live natural yogurt
sea salt and black pepper

Put the potatoes in a large saucepan and cover with cold water.
Bring to the boil and cook for about 15 minutes or until very
tender. Test with the tip of a knife.

   Heat the oil in a large saucepan and gently cook the spinach
leaves, garlic and spring onions for 2 minutes, stirring regularly
until softened. Set aside.

   Drain the potatoes in a colander and return to the saucepan.
Leave to stand for a couple of minutes. Mash the cooked potatoes
with the butter, milk and yogurt until smooth and season well to
taste. Use a set of electric beaters if you want your mash to be
really fluffy and light.

   Tip the spinach into the same pan and stir together over a
low heat until lightly combined and hot throughout. Transfer
to a warmed dish and serve. Drizzle with a little extra olive oil if
you like.

Simple vegetable stir-fry

Eat this simple stir-fry hot or cold with noodles. Get all the ingredients prepared before you begin to cook as it doesn't take long. Use your own mix of vegetables – it's a great way of using up odds and ends from the fridge. If planning to serve cold, adjust the initial cooking time to just 3 minutes, so the vegetables remain nice and crisp. Cool thoroughly and keep in the fridge. Eat within two days.

SERVES 2 | **PREP:** 10 minutes | **COOK:** 5 minutes

1 tbsp extra virgin olive oil
1 small red onion, peeled and cut into thin wedges
1 large carrot, peeled and thinly sliced
1 small red or yellow pepper, deseeded and thinly sliced

75g mangetout or sugar snap peas, trimmed
75g long-stemmed broccoli, trimmed and cut into short lengths
25g cashew nuts (optional)
1 tbsp dark soy sauce

Heat the oil in a large non-stick frying pan or wok and stir-fry the vegetables for 4–5 minutes or until just tender, adding the cashew nuts after 3 minutes. Season with the soy sauce and cook for a few seconds more.

MAKE A CHANGE
Look out for different-coloured vegetables, even vegetables such as carrots can come in a variety of different colours and will add diversity to your diet. If you see pak choi in your supermarket, slice thickly and add to the stir-fry too.

Bulgur wheat salad

This salad goes really well with Moroccan-inspired dishes and I serve it instead of couscous with tagines, spiced meats and fish as it's made with a prebiotic wholegrain that maintains its shape and texture without going soggy. It's also easy to transport for a gut-happy packed lunch. If you don't have all the different herbs, coriander alone will be almost as good.

SERVES 2 | **PREP:** 5 minutes | **COOK:** 10 minutes

75g bulgur wheat
1 lemon
2 tbsp extra virgin olive oil
1 garlic clove, peeled and crushed
bunch fresh coriander, leaves finely chopped (about 3 heaped tbsp)
15g fresh flat leaf parsley, leaves finely chopped (about 3 heaped tbsp)

10g fresh mint, leaves finely chopped (about 2 heaped tbsp)
3 spring onions, trimmed and finely sliced
20g pine nuts or flaked almonds
sea salt and black pepper

Half-fill a medium pan with water and bring to the boil. Add the bulgur wheat and cook for 8–10 minutes or until just tender, stirring occasionally. Cut the lemon in half and cut one half into four wedges. Squeeze the juice from the other half.

Drain the bulgur wheat in a sieve and press with the back of a spoon to squeeze out as much liquid as possible. Tip into a bowl and toss with the lemon juice, olive oil, garlic, coriander, parsley, mint, spring onions and pine nuts or flaked almonds.

Season with a little salt and lots of ground black pepper and toss well together. Serve with the lemon wedges for squeezing over the top.

MAKE A CHANGE
Finely grate a small orange and add the zest and juice to the salad.

Warm beans with garlic and lemon

A great alternative to potatoes, rice and pasta while bringing extra prebiotic fibre to any meal. You can use any beans you like – I generally choose white beans, such as cannellini, although borlotti are good too.

SERVES 2 | **PREP:** 5 minutes | **COOK:** 5 minutes

2 tbsp extra virgin olive oil
1 garlic clove, peeled and very
    thinly sliced
2 tbsp fresh lemon juice
400g can haricot or cannellini
beans, drained and rinsed
sea salt and black pepper
5g bunch flat leaf parsley, leaves
    finely chopped (optional)

Warm the olive oil with the garlic, lemon juice, a pinch of salt and lots of freshly ground black pepper in a medium saucepan over a low heat for a couple of minutes. Add the beans and heat gently for 1-2 minutes, stirring regularly until hot. Adjust the seasoning to taste and stir in some freshly chopped parsley if you like.

Dips, dressings and breads

I love the flexibility of this plan, the way you can mix and match different ingredients and come up with your own gut-healthy combinations. In the 28-day plan, you'll find different dips, dressings and breads cropping up. The dips are a great addition to your gut-happy platters. You can whizz them up in minutes, but they'll keep well in the fridge for up to three days. It's worth investing in a small food processor if you don't already have one – they're great for blitzing beans and other ingredients to make fantastic homemade dips.

I've included lots of probiotic yogurt here, and you'll find a range of dips made with prebiotic vegetables and pulses too. The dressings are for your salads and not surprisingly include plenty of olive oil, yogurt and garlic. Avoid shop-bought dressings as they often contain emulsifiers, thickeners and preservatives, many of which could disrupt your microbiome.

I've included a couple of breads here too. Mass-produced shop-bought bread usually contains various chemicals to improve shelf life, texture and rise, so if you can make your own you know exactly what is in it and how much fibre it contains and, your gut bacteria are likely to be a whole lot happier. If time is an issue, try to buy really good-quality bread from a more artisan producer, looking for sourdough ferments. Stay away from the highly processed sliced white breads and always choose wholegrain (wholemeal) bread, with a high fibre content, where you can.

The recipes

Homemade hummus

Feta and red pepper hummus

Artichoke and lemon dip

Olive oil vinaigrette

Balsamic vinaigrette

Yogurt mayonnaise

Blue cheese dressing

Yogurt flatbread

Wholemeal flatbreads

Homemade hummus

Tahini is an essential ingredient in this homemade hummus and is made with crushed sesame seeds. You'll find it in the world foods section of the supermarket and in many delicatessens.

SERVES 4-6 | **PREP:** 8-10 minutes

4 tbsp extra virgin olive oil
1 garlic clove, peeled and crushed
3 tbsp fresh lemon juice
400g can chickpeas, drained and
   rinsed

2 tbsp tahini (sesame seed paste
   from a jar)
4 tbsp cold water
sea salt and black pepper

Put the oil, garlic, lemon juice, chickpeas and tahini in a food processor. Add the water and salt and a few twists of freshly ground black pepper. Blend until as smooth as possible. You may need to remove the lid and push the ingredients down a couple of times until the right consistency is reached. Adjust the seasoning before serving.

Transfer to a small dish, cover the surface with clingfilm and keep covered in the fridge. Eat within 2 days. Serve with lots of fresh vegetable sticks.

FREEZING TIP

Freeze the hummus in small covered freezer-proof containers for up to one month. Thaw at room temperature for 2-3 hours before serving then stir well. Eat within two days.

Feta and red pepper hummus

This dish is perfect as a light lunch or supper, makes a useful packed lunch and, served with warm flatbread, is just the sort of thing you can put in the middle of the table for people to help themselves to. Use leftover feta for gut-happy platters or salads

SERVES 4 | **PREP:** 15–20 minutes | **COOK:** 10 minutes

1 tbsp extra virgin olive oil, plus extra for drizzling

1 large red pepper, deseeded and sliced into thin strips

1 large garlic clove, crushed

¼ tsp dried chilli flakes

400g can mixed beans, drained and rinsed

1 tbsp fresh lemon juice, plus 1 tsp

2 tbsp tahini (sesame seed paste)

65g feta cheese, drained

50g pitted olives (preferably Kalamata), drained

1 handful wild rocket leaves

2 tbsp mixed seeds, such as sunflower, pumpkin, sesame and linseed (flax)

sea salt and black pepper

warm flatbread, to serve

Put the olive oil in a small saucepan and place over a medium heat. Add the pepper, cover with a lid and cook for 10 minutes or until tender and lightly charred in places, stirring occasionally. (This will bring a subtle smoky flavour to the hummus.)

Add the garlic and chilli flakes to the pan and cook for a few seconds more, stirring constantly. Take off the heat and cool for 5 minutes. Put half the beans in a food processor, add the warm pepper, 1 tablespoon of the lemon juice and salt. Blitz until smooth.

Add the remaining beans, tahini and lots of ground black pepper and blitz until well combined but not quite smooth. Adjust the seasoning to taste, adding a little extra lemon juice or black pepper if needed. You don't need to add too much salt as the hummus will be topped with salty feta cheese. Scoop the hummus into a wide, shallow bowl and crumble the feta cheese over the top. Drizzle with olive oil.

Squish the olives lightly between finger and thumb and place in a bowl. Add the rocket leaves, remaining lemon juice and a few drops of olive oil. Toss very gently together then place on top of the hummus and feta and sprinkle with the mixed seeds. Put the dish on a platter or board.

Cut warm flatbread into wide fingers, place on the platter or board, with the feta hummus, drizzle with olive oil and serve.

Artichoke and lemon dip

An easy way to eat more artichokes and a great addition to a gut-happy platter. Keep in a lidded pot in the fridge for up to three days.

SERVES 4-6 | **PREP:** 10 minutes

390g can artichoke hearts (or 175g chargrilled artichoke hearts), drained
1 garlic clove, peeled
finely grated zest of ½ small lemon
1-2 tbsp fresh lemon juice
3 tbsp extra virgin olive oil
25g flaked almonds or mixed nuts, roughly chopped
sea salt and black pepper

Put the artichoke hearts, garlic, lemon zest, 1 tablespoon of the lemon juice, olive oil and almonds or mixed nuts in a food processor. Add a good pinch of salt and lots of ground black pepper. Blitz until well combined with a thick, dropping consistency. Adjust the seasoning to taste, adding a little extra lemon juice, salt and pepper if needed. Transfer to a small bowl.

Serve with vegetable sticks or warmed wholegrain or sourdough bread.

Olive oil vinaigrette

A classic dressing that goes well with any salad. Make a triple quantity of this dressing and it should last you at least 7 days. Pour into a clean jam jar after whisking, cover tightly and keep in the fridge. Give it a good shake before serving to recombine all the ingredients.

SERVES 4-6 | **PREP:** 5 minutes

1 tsp Dijon mustard
1 tsp caster sugar
2 tbsp red wine or cider vinegar

½ small garlic clove, peeled and crushed
8 tbsp extra virgin olive oil
sea salt and black pepper

Put the mustard, sugar, vinegar and crushed garlic in a bowl and season with a pinch of salt and some ground black pepper. Whisk with a metal whisk until well combined.

Gradually add the oil, whisking constantly until the dressing is thick. Adjust the seasoning to taste.

Balsamic vinaigrette

Serve this dressing with salads or drizzled over roasted vegetables. It's also a great seasoning to perk up Veggie bolognese and lasagne.

SERVES 4-6 | **PREP:** 5 minutes

1 tsp Dijon mustard
½ garlic clove, peeled and crushed
1 tbsp good-quality balsamic
  vinegar

4 tbsp extra virgin olive oil
sea salt and black pepper

Whisk the mustard with the garlic, balsamic vinegar, a good pinch of sea salt and lots of ground black pepper together in a bowl.

Slowly whisk in the olive oil until thickened and adjust the seasoning to taste.

Yogurt mayonnaise

A fab alternative mayonnaise made with lots of probiotic yogurt and polyphenol-rich olive oil. Use a full-fat live natural yogurt as it tastes richer and less acidic than the low-fat or fat-free versions and is likely to be better for you.

SERVES 4 | **PREP:** 5 minutes

100g full-fat live natural yogurt
½ tsp Dijon mustard
½ tsp red wine vinegar

½ tsp caster sugar
2 tbsp extra virgin olive oil
sea salt and black pepper

Mix the yogurt, mustard, vinegar and sugar in a small bowl and season with a pinch of salt and some ground black pepper.

Slowly stir in the oil until it is all incorporated. Adjust the seasoning to taste.

MAKE A CHANGE
Add a crushed clove of garlic to the mayonnaise for a fantastic aioli-style dressing – perfect for drizzling over roasted vegetables and Italian fish stew (page 201).

Blue cheese dressing

A simple cheese dressing, brimming with probiotic bacteria. If you add an extra 25g of cheese, it also makes a fantastic blue cheese dip – perfect for dipping celery sticks and chicory leaves or any other veg you fancy.

SERVES 2 | **PREP:** 5 minutes

25g Roquefort cheese, or other
   ideally unpasteurised (raw milk)
   blue cheese, rind removed
3 tbsp full-fat live natural yogurt

½ tsp red wine vinegar
1 tbsp extra virgin olive oil
black pepper

Mix together the cheese, yogurt and vinegar in a small bowl with a fork until well combined.

Slowly stir in the olive oil and mix until the sauce is glossy. Season to taste with ground black pepper. (You shouldn't need any salt as the blue cheese will be salty enough.) Transfer to a small bowl or drizzle directly over your salad.

Yogurt flatbread

This flatbread is very simple to make and tastes amazing. I've used a mixture of wholemeal and white flour to keep the bread light. Most of the live bacteria in the yogurt won't survive the cooking process but you will still benefit from the dairy content. Serve with curries, chillies and stews instead of rice, potatoes or pasta, for mopping up all the lovely sauce. Or add to your gut-happy platter.

MAKES 4 | **PREP:** 10 minutes, plus standing | **COOK:** 12–16 minutes

50g stoneground wholemeal plain flour, plus extra for rolling
150g self-raising white flour
½ tsp fine sea salt

100g full-fat live natural yogurt
3 tbsp warm water
1-2 tsp extra virgin olive oil, for greasing

Put both the flours and salt in a bowl and mix well. Add the yogurt and water and mix with a wooden spoon and then your hands to form a soft, pliable dough. Leave to stand for 5 minutes.

Divide the dough into 4 portions and roll out with a floured rolling pin on a well-floured surface into 4 roughly 18cm rounds, each about 4mm thick.

Grease a large non-stick frying pan with a little oil and place it over a medium–high heat. Cook the flatbreads, 1 at a time, for 1½–2 minutes on each side or until slightly risen and lightly browned. Keep warm, wrapped in a clean tea towel, while the rest are prepared.

FREEZING TIP
Freeze these breads in batches if you like. Wrap each one tightly in foil once cooled and freeze in a large labelled bag for up to one month. Reheat from frozen in a dry frying pan over a medium heat for 4–5 minutes, turning frequently, or in the microwave for 30–40 seconds, or until hot.

Wholemeal flatbreads

These wholegrain chapatti-like flatbreads are quick and easy to knock together. The method may look rather long, but I've added lots of detail in case you haven't made a flatbread like this before, and after you've made them the first time, you'll see how simple they are.

MAKES 2 | **PREP:** 5 minutes | **COOK:** 4–5 minutes

80g wholemeal plain flour, plus 10g extra for rolling
1 tsp extra virgin olive oil

3 tbsp warm water, plus a few drops if needed

Put the flour in a medium bowl and rub in the oil with your fingertips. Stir in the water and knead until the dough feels smooth and elastic, adding a few extra drops of water if necessary until the right consistency is reached.

Turn the dough onto a lightly floured surface and roll into 2 balls. Sprinkle the work surface with a little more flour and roll out 1 of the balls very thinly using a floured rolling pin. It needs to be around 22cm in diameter. Turn the dough regularly and sprinkle with a little more flour if it begins to stick. Put to one side and make the other flatbread in the same way.

Place a non-stick frying pan over a high heat and once it is hot, add one of the flatbreads. Cook for about 50 seconds, then turn over and cook on the other side for another 50–60 seconds. It should be lightly browned in patches and look fairly dry without being crisp. Press the flatbread with a spatula while cooking to encourage it to puff up and cook inside. Cook the remaining flatbread in the same way.

How to make the most of your freezer

When following the plan, you'll find that your freezer will soon become your best friend in the kitchen. You can not only buy frozen ingredients, such as berries and mixed vegetables, much more cost effectively when frozen, but you can keep home-cooked meals in the freezer ready to grab at a moment's notice. You'll save money on takeaway and restaurant meals and have the comfort of knowing there is always a nutritious, gut-friendly meal just minutes away.

- When freezing food, it's very important to allow it to cool rapidly after cooking. If you have made a casserole or curry, this means separating what you want to freeze from what you want to serve. Put in a shallow freezer-proof container, cover loosely and cool. Don't leave at room temperature for more than an hour. The shallower the container, the quicker the food will cool. (If you put it in the freezer while it is still warm, it will raise the temperature and could affect other foods.)

- If adding food that you have cooked in bulk for the freezer, make sure you flip the fast-freeze button on at least two hours before adding the new dishes and leave it on for twenty-four hours afterwards. The fast-freeze button will reduce the temperature of your freezer even further to help ensure that food is frozen as rapidly as possible.

- Cover food or wrap it tightly in a freezer bag or foil. It's vital to keep as much air out as possible. This will help prevent icy patches, freezer burn and discolouration and also stop flavours transferring between dishes whilst in the freezer. You should always leave a 2–3cm gap at the top of containers holding liquids as the liquid will expand on freezing.

- If you have a small freezer and need to save space, flat-freeze thick soups, sauces and casserole-style dishes in strong zip-seal freezer bags. Simply half fill the bag, then turn over and flatten until around 1–2cm thick, pressing out as much air as possible and sealing firmly. Foods frozen this way are really easy to cook from frozen too – just rinse the bag under hot water and break the mixture into a wide-based pan. Add a dash of water and reheat over a low heat until thawed. Increase the heat, adding a little more water if necessary, and simmer until piping hot throughout.

- Label everything going into the freezer well so you remember what you've added – not forgetting to write the date, so you know when to eat it at its best. I always try and use foods from the freezer within about four months as a slow deterioration will take place over time.

- Many foods can be defrosted slowly in the fridge for several hours or overnight. If you have flat-frozen foods (see above), it is far easier to cook from frozen as the dish will thaw and begin to reheat at almost the same time – my preferred method of preparing a quick meal. For safety's sake, do not thaw dishes at room temperature that you would normally keep in the fridge.
- Always ensure that any foods that have been frozen are thoroughly cooked or reheated before serving.

A few notes on the recipes

Ingredients

- Buy organic vegetables whenever you can.

- Where possible, choose organic and/or free-range chicken, meat and eggs. Eggs used in the recipes are medium unless otherwise stated.

- All poultry and meat has been trimmed of as much hard or visible fat as possible, although there may be some marbling within the meat.

- Boneless, skinless chicken breasts weigh around 150g. Fish has been scaled, gutted and pin-boned, and large prawns are deveined. You'll be able to buy most fish and seafood ready prepared, but ask your fishmonger if not and they will be happy to help.

Preparation

- Do as much preparation as possible before you start to cook. Discard any damaged bits, and wipe or wash fresh produce before preparation unless it's going to be peeled.

- Onions, garlic and shallots are peeled unless otherwise stated, and vegetables are trimmed. Lemons, limes and oranges should be well washed before the zest is grated. Weigh fresh herbs in a bunch, then trim off the stalks before chopping the leaves. I've used medium-sized vegetables unless stated. As a rule of thumb, a medium-sized onion and a potato (such as Maris Piper) each weigh about 150g.

- All chopped and sliced meat, poultry, fish and vegetable sizes are approximate. Don't worry if your pieces are a bit larger or smaller than indicated, but try to keep roughly to the size so the cooking times are accurate. Even-sized pieces will cook at the same rate, which is especially important for meat and fish.

- I love using fresh herbs in my recipes, but you can substitute frozen herbs in most cases. Dried herbs will give a different, more intense, flavour, so use them sparingly.

A word about puddings

If you love having a pudding and don't think any meal is complete without one, you may find adjusting to this plan a little tricky. I haven't suggested puddings in the 28-day menu plan, and it's ideal if you can resist. It's generally a good idea to get out of the habit of eating dessert after a meal as most puddings are high in saturated fat and sugar, both of which won't do your waistline or gut much good. An occasional sweet treat is fine but don't go mad.

If you are desperate for something sweet, go for a square of 70 per cent plus cocoa-solid chocolate. The flavour is so rich and satisfying that one piece should be enough. You can experiment with different dark chocolate from a variety of countries and also try chocolate with nuts and dried, or even freeze-dried, fruits for a change. You can help this down with some mint or herbal tea. And of course, don't forget about live yogurt – make your own combinations of natural bio yogurt and fresh fruit rather than buying fruit-flavoured or low-fat yogurts from the supermarket if you can. They are normally very high in sugar and often contain sweeteners and thickeners too. If you see a live fruit yogurt that has pectin as a thickener, choose it. Pectin is a great soluble fibre that is naturally found in fruit such as apples or pears, so you'll be increasing your prebiotic intake at the same time as benefiting from the probiotics in the yogurt.

General Index

5:2 diet 8
28-day plan 12, 13, 40, 70, 71, 74-81
   menus for 82-113
   frequently asked questions 116-123
   see also Recipe Index 305

acids, fatty 6, 20, 48, 49
alcohol 119, *see also* wine (red)
allergies 1, 3, 6, 8
Alzheimer's disease 75
anthocyanin 272
antibiotics 2, 3, 7, 41, 67, 74, 119, 123,
   151, 191
anti-inflammatories 49, 53, 272
antioxidant 6, 31, 32, 49, 51, 53, 57, 74
appendix 19
apple 6, 16-20, 25, 29, 37, 52, 56, 57,
   84, 127, 128, 132, 135, 301
artichoke *see* Jerusalem artichoke *or*
   globe artichoke
Asian cookery 7, 45, 71
asparagus 5, 25, 28, 29, 35, 127, 129,
   134, 135
aspartame 4

bacteria 7-9, 10, 16, 19, 20, 21, 22, 23,
   25, 26, 28, 29, 36, 38, 40, 41, 43,
   44, 45, 46, 47, 49, 53, 61, 67, 68,
   70, 114, 123, 135, 159, 173, 191, 207,
   208, 237, 242, 243, 246, 272,
   285, 295, 296
banana 5, 8, 26, 29, 36, 54, 118, 127,
   135
barley 29, 38, 58, 127
beans 5, 6, 10, 12, 23, 25, 26, 27, 29,
   32, 35, 36, 39, 52, 53, 58, 74, 79,
   80, 116, 117, 127, 131, 134
   canned 58, 120, 127, 131
beef 134, 173, 175
berries 6, 8, 43, 46, 51, 52, 54, 55, 57,
   60, 118, 127, 135
blood sugar control 21, 25, 38, 39,
   48, 52, 74

bowel 2, 20, 66
   diseases 21, 27
   the perfect poo 67-9
brain 13, 43, 63, 70
   chemicals 5
   function 20, 21
bread 7, 18, 26, 38, 44, 50, 60, 76,
   80, 116, 121, 127, 130, 132, 136, 285
breakfast 36, 37, 38, 42, 43, 44, 52,
   54, 59, 68, 75, 77, 118, 230, 233
breast milk 28
British Gut Project 10, 55, 114
brunch *see* breakfast
butyrate 6

C. difficile 2
calories 4, 6, 51, 52, 56, 59, 64, 65,
   119, 121, 128
cancer 6, 13, 37, 48, 55, 173, 207, 233
carbohydrates 18, 25, 26, 39, 104
cheese 4, 5, 7, 37, 41, 42, 43, 44, 45,
   50, 76, 80, 120, 121, 127, 128, 129,
   130, 132, 133
   unpasteurised 4, 5, 37, 42, 43, 44,
   50, 120, 127, 129, 130, 132, 133
chicken 8, 12, 50, 80, 121, 131, 134, 151,
   153, 300
chickpea 39, 52, 134
chocolate 6, 23, 48, 52, 53-4, 57, 81,
   96, 301
cholesterol 7, 16, 21, 25, 38, 39, 56
cocoa 6, 52, 53-4, 56-7, 301
coffee 6, 48, 56-7, 63, 64
colon 2, 5, 6, 7, 20, 49, 61, 67-9, 174,
   see also intestine (large)
constipation 66, 68, 69

dairy produce 7, 10
defrosting food 298-9
dementia 48, 55
depression, reducing 75
diarrhoea 20, 48, 67, 70, 123
dietary supplements 8

Recipe Index

Conversion tables

WEIGHTS & MEASURES

Tablespoon and teaspoon measures are level unless specified.
Note that in some recipes, liquids are weighed not measured in a jug.
A 'pinch' is as much as you can pick up with forefinger and thumb.
A handful – all you can grab. With herbs it is leaves only, not stalks.

CONVERSIONS

Weights: Metric – Imperial		Volume: Metric – Imperial	
5g	1/8 oz	1.25 ml	¼ tsp.
10g	¼oz	2.5 ml	½ tsp.
15g	½oz	5 ml	1 tsp.
25–30g	1oz	10 ml	2 tsp.
55g	2oz	15 ml	1 tbsp.
85g	3oz	30ml	2 tbsp/1 fluid oz
115	4oz	50 ml	2 fl oz
140g	5oz	60 ml	4 tbsp.
175g	6oz	100ml	3.5 fluid oz
200g	7oz	125ml	4 fluid oz
225g	8oz	200ml	7 fluid oz/⅓ pint
250g	9oz	300ml	10 fluid oz/½ pint
280g	10oz	500ml	18 fluid oz
350g	12oz	568ml	20 fluid oz/1 pint
375g	13oz	1 litre	1.75 pints
400g	14oz		
425g	15oz		
450g	1lb		
1kg	2lb 4oz		
2kg	4lb 8oz		

US Cups – Metric – Imperial

1 cup flour	150g	5oz
1 cup white sugar	225g	8oz
1 cup butter/lard	225g	8oz
1 cup ground almonds	110g	4oz
1 cup rice	200g	7oz
1 stick butter	110g	4oz

Acknowledgements

The first person I want to thank is my late father, John Pattison, a well-respected veterinary surgeon. As children, my brothers and I were never allowed to have antibiotics unless suffering from a life-threatening infection. We were encouraged to play with a variety of animals, benefited from an outdoor life and ate a varied diet (including his home-made yogurt). I am hugely grateful for such a fantastic start.

Massive thanks to Professor Tim Spector. Your ground-breaking book, *The Diet Myth*, made me rethink so much I thought I knew about food. I greatly appreciate all the guidance you gave me while writing this book – I hope I have done justice to all your research.

I'm truly grateful to the brilliant Claire Bignell for managing this project from my test kitchen. Your superb organisational and creative skills, combined with well-considered feedback has been crucial to its success.

Thanks to the very talented Angela Platt for her initial book designs, ideas and art direction and for creating such an amazing website for me. Emma Sturgess for her terrific research and for guiding and advising me on the more scientific aspects of the book; helping to keep everything simple. And my dear friend and physiotherapist, Tamsin Mann, for advice on all sorts of movements! And not forgetting photographer Cristian Barnett for the wonderful photographs that really make my menu plan come to life.

At Seven Dials, I am indebted to Amanda Harris for understanding what this book could mean to thousands of people. Also, thank you to Lucy Haenlein my lovely editor, for her guidance at the beginning, and the wonderful and meticulous Amy Christian for taking over the project and seeing it thorough to publication. Your eye for detail, reassuring manner and creative input has been invaluable.

Thanks also to Matt Inward for taking our rough layouts and turning them into a beautifully designed, very readable book. And for Helen Ewing for overseeing the design at every stage.

I'm also grateful to my agent, Zoe King, at The Blair Partnership, for her constant encouragement and enthusiasm. And the legal